Dear Kate

To Dear Ymenneth,

With my love and best
wishes.

Kate Sampson

Dear Kate

ALL THE ANSWERS TO YOUR PERSONAL PROBLEMS FROM AUSTRALIA'S BEST-LOVED ADVISER

Kate Samperi

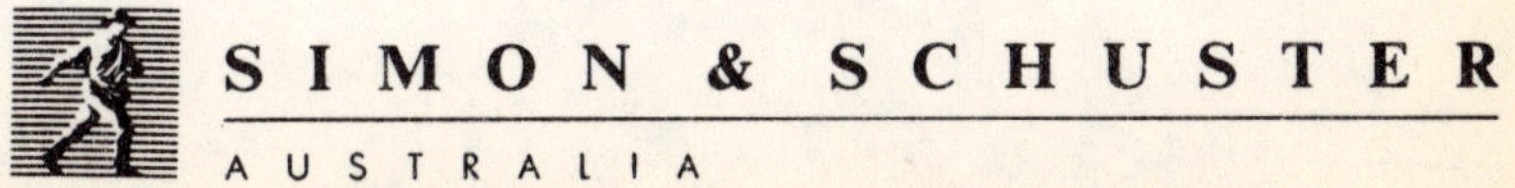

DEAR KATE: All the Answers to Your Personal Problems
from Australia's Best-loved Adviser

First published in Australasia in 1991 by
Simon & Schuster Australia
20 Barcoo Street, East Roseville NSW 2069

A Paramount Communications Company
Sydney   New York   London   Toronto   Tokyo   Singapore

National Library of Australia
Cataloguing in Publication data

Samperi, Kate.
   Dear Kate: all the answers to your personal
problems from Australia's best loved adviser.

   ISBN 0 7318 0228 4

   1. Women's day. 2. Newspapers — Sections, columns, etc.-
Advice. I. Title.

070.444

Designed by Michelle Havenstein.

Typeset in Garamond and American Typewriter by Excel Imaging.

Printed in Australia by Australian Print Group

Contents

6 HAVING AN AFFAIR   115

7 BEING SINGLE IN THE 90s   131

8 WHAT ABOUT SEX?   145

Introduction

ALL HUMAN BEINGS would like to be happy.

In the past 21 years I have read thousands of letters from people who have shared their innermost thoughts and feelings with me. Whatever the problem, the underlying request is always 'Please make me happy'. Most of them are in desperate situations, so desperate in fact, they are prepared to ask for help from an outsider in the hope that she will come up with some solution which they themselves cannot see. Often the solution is obvious, yet the person involved is too close to see it.

When people make a decision to write to me or consult another practitioner, it can be the turning point in their lives. By putting their thoughts on paper, they are putting space between themselves and their difficulties.

In many cases, what they focus on and write about is not the problem. They are seeing the symptoms but have no insights as to the cause. Yet the clues are always there. My area of expertise is to find those clues and then direct their attention to the aspects of the problem of which they are unaware.

Handling life successfully is looking with total honesty at our own behaviour, instead of blaming others when they don't respond the way we would like. We are always the ones projecting something which rebounds and hurts us.

This book is not intended as a cure-all for the multitude of human problems which beset us. But because I am privileged to hear so many secrets, I can identify those situations which seem to cause the most trouble for people. The letters in this book are just a few of the thousands I have read. They are representative, though, of the gamut of problems — the half-baked decisions, the unloving relationships, the lack of commitment — which people suffer. Although each problem is unique, it's a fact that most problems are common at least in part to all of us. There is comfort in knowing we are not alone, that there are others who struggle as we do. We can learn from one another.

By telling these stories about real people trying to cope with real problems, such as we all encounter in our day-to-day lives, I have tried to show how the way we behave is a reflection of the way we think about ourselves. Most importantly, how by changing our thoughts we *can* change our world if it is not working out the way we would like it to.

My hope is that the letters and my responses which follow will act as a kind of therapy for those who read them. In reading how other people are mishandling their lives, we can hold up a mirror for ourselves and recognise something of our own predicament. At such times it's a good idea to ask ourselves: 'Is this me? Do I behave like that?' This can give us insight into what we are doing in a practical way.

Problems are an opportunity for growth, and in accepting the challenge to face the problems, we give ourselves the chance to improve our lives.

As we correct each false idea about ourselves, we experience a move toward a less complex and more balanced way of looking at life. What is rewarding is that once we start on this course, the quality of our life and the feelings we have about ourselves improve from that moment on. We start to have hope, things make more sense, solutions are possible and we feel more confident in meeting the difficulties which face us.

I have seen many changes in these 21 years, but two things have remained constant — the resilience of the human spirit, and our innate desire for fulfilment and happiness. This has led to a burgeoning interest in self-knowledge, in learning new ways to make our lives richer. More and more people are embarking on this fascinating journey.

So join me now in this exploration of human behaviour. Who knows, we may break through a few barriers of our own . . .

Kate Sampson

SYDNEY 1991

1
Self-esteem

'SELF-ESTEEM' HAS BECOME one of the catchwords of the eighties and it is used glibly and often to explain everything that goes wrong in a person's life from blushing to poor relationships. Where years ago people wrote about their 'inferiority complex', they now talk about their low self-esteem.

Self-esteem is how we feel about ourselves, how much we like who we are and how glad we are to be this person called 'me'. We recognise its importance when we see that from our earliest years, our attitude towards ourself has a direct bearing on the friends we choose (or who choose us), how we get on with others, the use we make of our abilities, and even the kind of person we marry. It affects how we think and feel and whether or not we shall make a success of life.

Early on we get an idea about ourselves from the way our parents, teachers and anyone else influential in our lives reacts towards us. Because our minds are young and impressionable at that age, the feelings their comments and attitudes engender stay with us. If we cling to these beliefs as we get older, we perceive everything that happens to us through the eyes of the child we were, instead of in the context of our adult life.

In general, the person with low self-esteem has received more negative than positive messages in childhood and through life. Many people are programmed to believe 'You're never good enough', and go through life feeling they have failed, no matter what their achievements. Parents rarely set out to harm their children intentionally. But if they themselves had misleading

1

and damaging messages from their parents, it is likely that they are still passing them on. Their lack of knowledge and awareness perpetuates the same problems in their children.

This new realisation that self-esteem is vital to our emotional wellbeing, is a healthy sign. The term itself is more positive than the old term, 'inferiority complex', which implied no possibility of change. With self-esteem you can progress from 'low' to 'high' and this is the goal of the many courses being run by trained counsellors. The waiting list for these courses is always long. I often recommend such courses and advise those of you wanting to improve your own self-esteem to enquire at a community health centre as to what is available in your local area.

I FEEL INADEQUATE

Janice wrote:

> 'Ever since I can remember I have never felt at ease
> with people I don't know very well. I feel I don't
> measure up to their standards, that I am not as
> interesting, not as poised, and I go over any
> conversation we've had and could kick myself for what
> I said. Then I magnify it until I blush with shame at
> my inadequacy. If anyone looks at me, I always think
> they are noticing all the faults in my appearance. But
> the strangest thing is that today one of my work
> colleagues said she envied me my confidence and calm
> manner! If only she knew ... !'

'Maybe she doesn't know, but neither do you, that everyone, from beautiful actors to timid clerks, all suffer from feelings of insecurity', I replied. 'It takes many forms, of course. Some people feel inferior, some are anxious, shy, apprehensive, or too eager to please. It may even take the form of being superior and aloof — the man who boasts of his success with women is really admitting his failure to form lasting relationships. And the girl who may be accused of looking down her nose at others, is really afraid of relating to other people.

'We all try to cover our inadequacies as best we can, always wishing we were as beautiful/intelligent/cool/poised as someone else, while they envy us our serenity. The truth is that nobody is completely confident in all areas all of the time. When you admit this fact to yourself, you are taking the first step towards conquering your feelings of inadequacy. Remember that self-confidence begins with your own attitude and you can choose your attitude: will you expect to fail or be ineffectual, or will you see yourself as dynamic, talented, attractive, and successful? The choice is yours and what you see in your mind's eye over a period of time is what you will become. To know we have such power within ourselves should be one of the greatest confidence boosters imaginable. And I assure you it works. When you succeed, tell yourself you're pretty marvellous. When you have an occasional setback, tell yourself you're pretty wonderful because you're trying — which makes you a terrific person all the time.'

Lisa sounded as if she was about to give up on herself:

'I hope to heaven you can help me find out why everything I do turns to mud. If I have friends to dinner no one seems to enjoy it and they leave early. If I am on any project or committee, bang!, it's total disaster. I seem to be a walking jinx! Yet I always try so hard to do the right thing, and I'm sick with anxiety beforehand to make things work out. So why don't they? I might add the reason I am fed up is because I have suffered in this way since I was a child and I can't stand myself much longer.'

'If everything you do is jinxed,' I answered, 'it's because you expect it to be so. The crux of your problem is the fact that you don't like yourself. And as with everyone we meet, all that we do is affected by the way we feel about ourselves. It is this self-image which determines how we respond to the world around us and how it reacts to us, whether we make our own good or bad luck. It is the core of our personality and it governs every aspect of our behaviour, from our choice of friends, life partners and careers, to our capacity to learn or to grow and change. Unfortunately, after repeated failures, we develop a self-perpetuating pattern of poor performances. This is what has happened to you.

'Before we can like anyone else we must like ourselves and by your own admission, you can't stand yourself any longer. I doubt you would ever be so cruel to any other person. Learn to like yourself and the rest of your world will follow. Begin by writing down a list of all the good things about yourself: they don't have to be *big* virtues. Just ordinary little things you take for granted in yourself. You'll find the list is longer than you had thought possible at first. Then write down all the qualities you'd like to possess — confidence, for instance, optimism, humour . . . Concentrate on examples you can think of for each of these qualities several times a day and last thing before you go to sleep so your subconscious can do its work. See yourself as already possessing these qualities.

Stop being a stick-in-the-mud and stretch your mind with challenges beyond the limits imposed by routine. Learn to react to life's circumstances in a positive way. The way you see yourself is what you will become.'

The ability to see ourselves as others see us — not better, not worse, but just as we are — is a useful attribute and a rare one. Rachel's letter illustrates this point:

'I am a young college student who is very lonely. No matter what opportunities come up and what efforts I make, I never seem to make good friends with anyone, least of all with boys. I have a few acquaintances I've met through college, work and gatherings but they all seem to be tied up with their own lives and friends and I back off feeling unwanted, pretending everything is fine when it is not. I used to have a small group of four friends and we were very close, but now we have drifted apart, not from my choice.

'If I were arrogant, obnoxious or rude, I would understand why people don't like me, especially boys. However, I consider myself a warm, open, friendly, giving person. I am not critical and don't expect much from others. I believe a good friendship is something that will or won't develop and has a lot of give and take. I've been on anti-depressants for this problem as sometimes I get overwhelmed with feelings of inadequacy and loneliness. I'm starting to avoid social gatherings because even though I try to fit in with the crowd and enjoy myself, I usually end up sitting in a quiet corner or going home early.

'I feel as if there's a great void in my life. I can't express my deep feelings of loneliness and unhappiness but hope you understand. I want to have friends and to be a good friend. And I would like to have a boyfriend. Can you help me?'

I was glad Rachel had written such a long, honest letter — it must have done her good to write down her deepest feelings and given her a clearer perspective of what her problem was.

'I'm sure you are warm, friendly and giving, all of which should make it easy for you to make friends of both sexes,' I wrote back. 'But somehow, these are not the qualities which you exhibit. What comes through is your desperate loneliness, your poor self-esteem and your feelings of helplessness. You have no sense of self and are too eager to please. You don't expect much and that is exactly what you are getting. All this is bound to turn people away because it makes them uneasy. They have enough insecurities of their own and can't stand anyone else's. They prefer people who are confident and cheerful and enthusiastic, because it activates their own positive energy. It is clear to me you are a sensitive, thinking person who would be good company if she could be with like-minded young people. At present, all your good qualities go unnoticed because you are so self-effacing.

'Before you can be a good friend to anyone you must first of all be a good friend to yourself. We can only give out from ourselves and not from a deficit sense of need. Your depression is a sign that there are things in your life you'd rather not look at and it also means your energy is blocked like a stagnant pool. Take up some activity which will get your energy moving again and this will be reflected in your mental outlook as well.

'Don't avoid social gatherings but don't go there with great expectations. Just be part of them in your own quiet way. You don't have to feel a failure because you are not the life of the party. And try to mix with different groups, so that you have a broader choice. The best group for you to join would be one where you are working towards a common goal, as well as enjoying social activities. In the process of working together you make good friendships. ROTORACT, a group with Rotary for young people, is such an organisation and is nationwide.

'And why not invest in a self-development course? That would help you find out what makes people tick and improve your relationships. It is also a good place to meet people who are seeking deeper truths as you are and so you would have something in common from the very start.'

Modern men are often accused of lacking commitment but the next letter from Leanne shows it can affect women just as much.

'I am 20 years old and still don't know what I want out of life. I'm in love with a 27-year-old man who doesn't want any kind of commitment to me or anyone else. I don't want a commitment either. In fact, I've never had a relationship lasting more than a few months. All I want is someone to love me but not be there every day. I know it's because I have low self-esteem and constantly feel insecure, but I lack the confidence to seek help. I don't have a job and feel as if my life is simply slipping away. I feel like a total mixed-up mess.'

'Your description of yourself sounds very apt. The way you perceive life is out of kilter and what you need is good counselling to unfog your vision. To begin with you need to know that commitment is a source of joy, and having no commitment is to be partially dead. If that is how you want to spend the rest of your life, that's your great loss. Otherwise take yourself by the scruff of your neck and make some changes which will turn your life around and make it worth living. People are most miserable when their attention is anchored on themselves, so join a group, a class, a cause — anything which will open your vision to what is outside yourself and claims your interest.

'Contact your nearest CES office. Even if you can't find a job, they have many programmes and activities to improve your skills and make you feel causative. Check your nearest Community Health Centre or local council to find out what is available, including self-development classes and counselling facilities. Objective, professional help will help you overcome your difficulties.'

I receive more letters from women than men. But this one from Bob is typical of many from both sexes, which shows that both men and women can suffer from the same anxieties.

> 'My problem is making me miserable and moody, so I hope you can help me. I always feel I am not as good as other people. For example, when in a group I suddenly wonder why people would want to be talking to me, and feel they are probably finding me boring and only put up with me because I work with them. That's why I'm scared to ask a girl to go out with me. She would probably say 'no' because I am not much to look at and can't carry on an interesting conversation. Tell me, Kate, how can I overcome these feelings, as I know they are ruining my life?'

'The only thing that can make you inferior is thinking you are inferior', I said. 'It's a well-known fact that we end up becoming what we think we'll be. It even has a name — the self-fulfilling prophecy — so you see I'm not just saying it to make you feel better. Our minds are like computers — the results are based on the information we feed into them. If you feed in "I'm inferior", your subconscious will make you behave in that way even when you're not aware of it. But if you feed in: "I'm a worthwhile person. I am interesting. I can make things happen", that is exactly what you *will* do.

If at present you are dull and uninteresting, whose fault is it? And who is the only person who can change all that? Right then, stop moaning and start acting! Take up hobbies and interests, read all you can, get into discussions with friends, listen as well as talk, and reach out to other people. You are probably more interesting than you give yourself credit for being (boring people are rarely aware that they are boring), but you simply haven't given yourself a chance. If a girl says "no" to your request, it isn't the end of the world, nor does it mean you are at fault. There are lots of young women out there trying to meet men. You just try again and again. Give your "computer" some worthwhile facts to work on. The results may jolt you into discovering your real potential.'

Marie's letter was interesting because it gives a clear picture of what self-esteem really is. It is being who we are, not what other people think we ought to be.

> 'My husband and I have completely different personalities — he is out-going and full of fun, and I am quiet and shy. Whenever we go to a party or any occasion where there are a lot of people, he has a wonderful time, but for me it's agony. I can't find anything interesting to say so I clam up and stand there like a prize idiot, trying to look as if I'm alive, but all I'm waiting for is the time my husband says "Let's go home". He says I should try harder to be bright, but the more he says it, the worse I am. I think if I didn't have to try to be what I'm not, I could cope better.'

'Your last sentence sums up a very important truth: that unless we can be ourselves we end up being nobody at all,' I replied. 'I know this is not as easy as it may first appear. Most of us are obliged to operate behind a façade at least part of the time. We have to adapt to people and situations, to behave and speak and smile in the way we think is expected of us. But there's a limit. If you are an introvert, why should you play the extrovert? The energy you expend trying to be what you are not is enormous. And why do you believe that the life of the party is superior to a quieter person?

Accept the fact that there is a place for bright, lively people and a place for quiet, shy ones and that each has a part to play in any worthwhile relationship. This acceptance of yourself will in itself give you more confidence and will draw others to you. There is something comforting about people who are calm and serene and make no demands on others to be anything but themselves. There are too few of them. Please your husband by showing him you have some spirit: tell him to belt up! Then go on being yourself.'

Helen's letter tells us more about her husband's low self-esteem than hers which she believes is the problem. She wrote:

'I am married to an intellectual with a strong
personality. I think he feels he married beneath him.
He rubbishes so much of what I do and often puts me
down when our friends visit us, and when we are
alone, he is always buried in books as if I didn't exist.
My only use to him seems to be in bed. But I love him
and think he loves me. I just wish I wasn't so inferior
to him — my level of education is not as high as his,
but I am good at other things and our friends seem to
like and respect me. Can you help me?'

'You have allowed yourself to be dominated by your husband', I replied, 'not because you *are* inferior to him, but because you have convinced yourself that you are. His own self-esteem must be pretty shaky, and he needs to put you down in order to build himself up. Of course, you have gone along with his game by behaving like a mouse, nervous in case you disturb the master-mind around the house. I'll bet you have never expressed an opinion of your own in case he disagrees. Let him disagree! That is healthy communication. What is unhealthy is if you slink around the place afraid to put a foot or a word wrong. You have come to regard him as some kind of supreme being just because he's got a little more than average keeping his ears apart.

'Come now, where is your commonsense? Find it quickly. If he puts you down when friends are around it's because he's got the silent message you've been giving him, which is: 'If I open my mouth, I'm sure to disgrace you.' Tell yourself you are his equal and his superior, sometimes, in other ways. I bet he knows it, too. The important thing is that *you* realise it. Your friends are giving you feedback that it's true.'

Shirley's letter expresses what many women feel:

'I don't believe in myself, and realise now that is why
nobody else does. I'm 28 years old, and over the past
10 years my only achievements in life are my husband
and three children. I never get any encouragement to

> take on a new idea — my husband seems happy letting
> me hang on to my low self-esteem. And yet I am really
> an excellent wife and mother, qualities which
> continually go unnoticed. Probably my story is similar
> to so many others, but what advice can you give me?'

I had to agree that there are many women with a similar story, yet could not go along with her blaming her husband for her lack of motivation. No one outside ourselves can inspire us, unless we are already inspired. Often it is easier to use someone 'out there' as an excuse for not changing.

'Perhaps he is not as demonstrative as you would like, but the fact that he accepts you as you are is a compliment in itself and should boost your good feelings about yourself,' I said.

I urged her to do something different — a course of study, a craft, learning a musical instrument, a discussion group, or even a stint of charity work where she would come into contact with other women, all of which would boost her confidence and sharpen his interest. The routine of everyday life can dull any marriage, and deaden any woman's self-esteem. It is up to each individual to work at both the marriage and the self-esteem. 'There are no limits to what you can do unless you put them there yourself,' was my parting reply.

THE BORN JOKER

Sylvia's letter did not seem to fit the usual picture of the person suffering low self-esteem. I imagine that on the surface she might even appear to have high self-esteem. However, all the clues were there.

> 'I'm 18 and have just started working and am very
> happy. My problem is that I don't think I like myself. I
> make friends very easily, mainly because I am a born
> joker. But people cannot understand that I have a
> serious side, so that when I am depressed I can't
> explain how I feel because I am usually so happy. I am
> rather overweight, supposedly pretty, but can't gain
> any confidence. It doesn't worry me much that I
> haven't a boyfriend as I have plenty of 'boy' friends at

work, but now that I have matured considerably (since beginning work), I could handle a one-to-one relationship. Not a sexual one though, as I have fairly religious views on the matter. Some days I feel so boring, unloved and stupid, and on other days I feel worthwhile and that I am getting more attention than I deserve. Deep down I suppose I sort of like myself, but I just want to feel more confident and wanted. I hope you can give me some direction in overcoming my problem.'

I sensed that Sylvia, like most of us, was a mixture of high and low self-esteem. Basically she seemed to have some self-respect and a belief in her own convictions, which is the basis for building self-esteem. She has a clear picture of herself as being attractive to the opposite sex and does not sell herself short in this respect. The fact that she has lots of friends of both sexes is also an indication that she projects a pleasing personality.

Her lack of self-confidence is to be taken in the context of her age. Most 18-year-olds wish they had more confidence although not all would admit it. What is sabotaging Sylvia is her feeling that she is not reaching anybody from her *real* self. Her real self is rarely allowed to come out because of her own doubts. She is never sure when she has been accepted by people. Her judgement is impaired, so she keeps trying and ends up with overkill. How can people see her serious side if she is hiding behind the mask of the joker? I felt it was her way of not getting too close to her real self. Full-time jokers are not always motivated by happy feelings — they do it because they want to please and feel they can't do it any other way.

At the same time they are putting themselves down by playing the clown, they resent the fact that no one will take them seriously. I felt that Sylvia was so busy keeping up a front out of fear she might not be liked, that she never allowed herself to be who she really is. No wonder she gets depressed. All that effort is exhausting. My advice to her was to 'let go' of all her acting and accept herself as a good and worthwhile person with many of the frailities which make her human just like the rest of us. I felt she had the willingness to grow and develop in the future, and the potential to develop a high self-esteem.

THE COMPULSIVE CHATTERER

The next letter from Jodie shows an unexpected side of low self-esteem.

'Is there such a thing as a compulsive chatterer? Although I make up my mind I'm not going to tell people my problems and things, the next thing I know, I've told them everything about myself. I'm not a gossip, but I can't help revealing things I'd rather keep to myself. It's got me into trouble a few times and I know my friends don't take me seriously because of it. The worst part is that I feel so dreadful after I've gabbed, but it's as if I can't stop myself.'

Compulsive talking is usually a sign of low self-esteem, of nervousness and anxiety. The talkative person (in this case Jodie) tries to make other people like her by 'giving' information about herself and other people as a kind of 'gift'. This is also an attempt to manufacture intimacy and friendship. In fact, this need can cause them to gossip and results in people mistrusting them.

Jodie's letter illustrates how lack of self-respect destroys self-esteem. Each time she gave in to her compulsive behaviour she 'felt dreadful'.

The only way Jodie can overcome this problem is to begin liking herself and to be as kind and tolerant to herself as she would be to anyone else. Then she would have no need to give away all that she owns and that includes her own private knowledge. The first time Jodie stops herself from 'gabbing', her self-esteem will be on the way up. She will no longer have to act out her 'please love me' tape, which is covering up her feeling that she is unlovable.

I pointed out that since she was already aware that her problem was painful, disturbing and destructive to her relationships with others, she had a head start in finding solutions. I suggested that if she could not find solutions on her own, professional help was advisable.

BEAUTY IS *NOT* SKIN-DEEP

The way we look, or the way we *think* we look, is important to all of us, but for teenagers it can be a source of despair. Consider this letter from Debbie:

'Because I am rather overweight, I lack confidence in myself. I am in my mid-teens and have never had a boyfriend. I tend to think that guys don't want to be seen with me as a girlfriend as they might be too embarrassed by my being overweight. I know that if a guy really did care he wouldn't worry about how much weight I carry, but are there guys like that? I have dieted many times but find it hard to lose weight. I am not at all pretty and this is always on my mind. Mum thinks I'm attractive and that I'll be beautiful as I get older. But all the guys at school call me a dog and if the guys think that, I must be ugly. How can I possibly grow to be pretty when I am so ugly now? I try to be happy and cheerful and not worry about things but it doesn't help and it doesn't work. Am I always going to be rejected because I am not pretty and slim? Isn't it what's on the inside that counts or will I always be judged by my weight?'

Debbie's plea touched me and I wished I could be like Cinderella's fairy godmother and wave a magic wand.

'Of course it's the person we are inside that counts,' I replied, 'and more than most of us imagine. It's a fact that the way we feel about ourselves deep down, the image we have of who we are, affects all our relationships and even the way we look on the outside. If we think we are ugly, we somehow project ugliness. Unless we like ourselves first, we can't really like anyone else and it's odds on they won't like us.'

People take their cues on how to treat us from the way we treat ourselves. I urged her to begin a little image therapy. I asked her to imagine how she'd like to be and then work at seeing it come about. 'See yourself as a warm, humorous, loving and lovable person and that is what you will become.'

Because Debbie rejects herself so much, she expects to be rejected by guys, and so she puts out vibes which bring about what she is afraid of. What Debbie needs to know is that at this age, boys also have a shaky self-esteem and need to go with the prettiest, most popular girl with the best figure in order to boost their own lack of self-confidence. They need a prop to make them feel 'cool'. And they don't have the insight and awareness that there is more to a girl than a pretty face and a good shape. It takes maturity to know these things.

Another fact which Debbie is not aware of is this: her fear of being rejected by boys keeps her locked into remaining fat. If she feels she is not worth much, why bother trying to be attractive? It is easier to blame the extra pounds for all her problems than to look for what else may need changing. It becomes a vicious circle: while she is feeling wretched she will undoubtedly find consolation in food, thus perpetuating her problem.

I suggested that if Debbie had not read the story of the Ugly Duckling she should go and read it at once. I also pointed out that she was lucky to have such a wise and understanding mother to stand by her during this difficult part of her adolescent development.

Even if Debbie doesn't grow up to be an archetypal beauty, by whose standards will she be judged? Tastes in looks have changed through the centuries and every society and culture sees beauty through a different lens. The poet, Keats, said it perfectly when he wrote: 'Beauty is in the eye of the beholder'.

Anna wrote:

> 'My problem is that I'm not very pretty so my
> boyfriend is ashamed to take me out. We used to go out
> a bit in the afternoons when his mates were at work,
> but after we saw his ex-girlfriend who's very pretty, he
> stopped taking me out altogether. Now we just meet at
> my house. He says he loves me and that when we move
> interstate together it will be different, but I wonder if
> he means it. We're both 16.'

'No matter where you go, it won't be different', I replied. 'The problem is between the two of you. You are both young and filled with insecurities. He needs a pretty girlfriend to bolster his low self-esteem and your worries, which are normal at your age, would disappear if you had a loving boyfriend you made you *feel* pretty. By treating you as an ugly secret, he's destroying all your self-confidence. Tell him this. It might make him change. If it doesn't, find yourself another boyfriend who will appreciate you just as you are. But please don't make any hasty plans to move away with him before you sort things out.'

Teenagers are not the only ones made unhappy by their looks. Consider this letter from Beryl:

'I am 42 and after staying home for twenty years to rear my family, I have gone back to work after a period of training. I am happy and excited at what promises to be a good career, but my problem is that the oldest girl in my group is 25 and I feel so old. These girls seem to have so much fun out of life! I wish I could join them but I am not the type.

'The funny thing is that I have always felt old even when I was young. I was the eldest in my family and even as a child I remember being much older and more staid than the others even though there were only two years between us. My mother used to call me her "right-hand man" and I loved helping her, but sometimes I wished she'd hug me the way she did my two younger sisters. But she never did. I'm sure she loved me but she always treated me as if she and I were the same age. Now I'm fed up with being old! Can you give me the name of a good cosmetic surgeon so that I can get rid of a few wrinkles and gain a lot of confidence by getting a "younger" face?'

As the eldest child, Beryl would have been given responsibility beyond her years. With two younger children to care for it would have been easy for her mother to overlook the fact that Beryl, like all children, also needed affection. On one level Beryl was proud of being her mother's helper and even played her part in spoiling the little ones. Yet on another level it hurt her that she was always expected to be the sensible one, the serious older sister, the one who didn't mind going without if there wasn't enough. In a later letter she confirmed that she was always expected to behave like an adult and never like a child not even when she was six or seven years old. She yearned to be mothered and cuddled, but her mother was always too busy with the others. I guessed that after her marriage, Beryl would have been a mother who gave too much to her children, trying to be the mother she had always wanted but did not have.

What was Beryl really afraid of now? She sounded ambitious, attractive and interesting, and she had the experience which comes through living, as well as the experience gained through marriage and rearing a family. I was sure the girls she worked with admired these qualities.

In the correspondence which ensued with Beryl, I reminded her that no matter how much mothering we had in our earlier years, most of us wish we had more. For those who were really deprived or *thought* they were deprived, there was a deficit in their lives which nothing seemed to fill. As adults they could try to get this mothering from a spouse or lover, and from warm, nurturing friendships, but the main source now would have to come from themselves. This is not as self-centred as it sounds, for unless we can nurture ourselves we are unable to nurture anyone else. I urged Beryl to be kind to herself, to treat herself as she would a beloved friend, to nurture the child in her which had grown up too quickly, to mother it in the way she had wanted to be mothered back then. She could do this by giving herself treats occasionally, by indulging herself in doing something she really wants to do — having a perfumed bubble bath for instance, or a special salon facial or massage. Or she can buy something she wants but would not normally buy. It can be as expensive as a glamorous dress or as minimal as a bunch of violets or a luxury magazine.

The message Beryl keeps hearing is 'be responsible' which means doing for other people. She can help reverse this by allowing others to do things for her, and even asking for what *she* wants. If and when the younger people in her office ask her to join them in their fun-times she should join them instead of pulling back. It would do her the world of good.

I also suggested that if she really was serious about cosmetic surgery, she should first indulge in some special clothes, a new hairstyle and some make-up. In her last letter to me she said she had taken up walking for half an hour each morning and was already feeling trim and alive. She still had not made up her mind about cosmetic surgery, but had splurged on clothes and had a whole new look. She admitted that she liked the way the younger girls in the office looked up to her and sought her advice about their love lives. She ended her letter with the words: 'Being an older sister has its compensations.' I knew then that Beryl had begun to accept herself.

I CAN NEVER SAY 'NO'

Many people can identify with the next letter from Mary:

'My problem is that I can never say "no". No matter what I am asked to do and how inconvenient it is for me, I always give in. Then I could kick myself for being so weak, but by then it's too late. It's not that I want to be aggressive or mean, but I feel I am always being taken advantage of and want to change it.'

I was certain Mary had never said 'No, I don't want to do this or that' to anyone. I assured her it was about time she did and that it would be easier each time she practised it.

'There's no need to give a reason as to why you're saying "no" unless it happens to be someone close to you, in which case you may want to give some sort of explanation to avoid offending them,' I advised. 'But don't let yourself be manipulated either by criticism or guilty feelings, or by anyone assuming he or she knows what is best for you.'

Most importantly, she should refuse to let others make her responsible for their problems so that they can manipulate her into doing what they want her to do. It is possible she would not feel confident to say 'no' or be impervious to others' opinions, but paradoxically, each time she does stand up for herself, her confidence and belief in her own worth will be strengthened. And each time she is weak and gives in, her confidence will be further undermined. I reminded her that we can't be loved by everybody and that if we keep on saying yes when we really mean no, we end up playing a role and expending tremendous energy in trying to fool ourselves and other people. We end up being liked by nobody. At least, if we like ourselves there is somebody on our side!

SELF-ESTEEM AND SEX

All the letters so far illustrate some aspect of low self-esteem which affects the writers' lives and relationships to varying degrees. The next letter from Janet, however, gives a more destructive picture:

> 'I'm 20 and for the past three years have gone out with at least twelve men. My problem is that I can never say 'no' when they ask for sex. If anything, I want them to ask me. I didn't worry about this until recently I met a very special boy and fell in love with him. I'm almost certain he feels the same way about me. If he asks me to marry him — which I think he will — I'd hate for him to find out I'm a nymphomaniac and I couldn't bear to let him down because of my weakness.'

Janet is no nymphomaniac. What she doesn't know is that when a girl has sex with any man who asks her, it always means she has a desperately low opinion of herself. Feeling she is not lovable and has nothing to offer except her body, she gives it compulsively. In complying with men's demands she is selling herself cheap for a few moments of closeness with another human being. This is too high a price to pay. Each time she gives in, her feelings of self-worth are damaged even more, so every time she jumps into bed in an effort to convince herself and everyone else that she is attractive and desirable and lovable, the end result is the very opposite.

By taking on the label of nymphomaniac, Janet is doing herself untold damage. When we label ourselves a certain way we subconsciously make sure we act out the role we have chosen. I told her that it is not sexiness which motivates her promiscuity but her deep feelings of insecurity.

CHRONIC BLUSHING

Tom's problem is one I have heard often since I first began my column. It is a problem which never goes away completely.

'I am an 18-year-old boy and suffer from chronic
blushing. I used to think I'd grow out of it, but now
I'm getting desperate. I can't do things I want to
because of my fear of blushing. It's ruining my life.'

'What is it that is frightening you so much and ruining your
life?' I wanted to know. 'Simply a red face, and a red face isn't
that important. The only way to get rid of this problem is to stop
thinking of it as a problem. Some people sweat when they're shy,
some talk too much, some stammer and others do their best to
become invisible. And we're all shy sometimes! What is silly is to
double the shyness by worrying about the effect of shyness. If
you do that, you get even redder, and that makes you even more
shy, which makes you redder and so on and so on. It's up to you
to break the chain by ignoring the shyness and the blushing.'

2

Marriage

SOME YEARS AGO I read an anecdote about marriage which made me smile. 'Marriage,' it said, 'is like a besieged fortress, with those outside madly trying to get in and those inside desperately trying to get out.'

At the time it amused me. Today it may be closer to the mark than we'll admit.

In the early years of my column, marriage was still the 'done' thing. Then came the sexual revolution and the rumblings of discontent began. We looked at marriage with critical eyes and found it wanting. Many reasons have been suggested for this decline in family life — greater sexual freedom, freedom of choice, women entering the workforce in the sixties and seventies, and the breakdown of some social traditions.

I remember the many letters from working mothers racked with guilt that they were neglecting their children. The debates on this topic were endless, the solutions conflicting.

Yet disquieting as they are, these changes are not a new or sudden phenomenon. Marriage has changed and evolved and survived for many centuries, keeping up with and reflecting other social changes.

For centuries marriage was a business arrangement between families, a contract and obligation with no talk of choice or love. Romantic love as a basis for marriage came much later as a revolt against such impersonal, soulless mating. The romantic era introduced the gentler, more noble aspects of love and living-happily-ever-after. But then came the Victorian era, and with it, a great deal of repression and guilt.

The Victorian rigidity of thought and feeling began to break down during the first World War and later during the Second World War when women went to work for the war effort and discovered new freedoms and latent capabilities. The seeds of the much later sexual revolution were sown then.

Yet despite the many changes and its unstable image, marriage is still popular and regarded as the ideal for the majority. Why then is it often more disappointing and subject to disruption than in the past?

I believe one of the main reasons is that we expect too much of it. We rely on it to satisfy many emotional needs which were once satisfied by a network of close relationships. The Nuclear Family was a big reaction to the huge families in Victorian times. For a while it was considered the ideal, but as with all innovations, its deficiencies did not take long to appear.

We all gain from sharing with a large number of people. The Nuclear Family was a form of isolation in which we expected all our satisfactions to come from one source — our partner. In those years I saw many marriages break under the strain, with husbands leaving home and family, and wives suffering unending depression and breakdowns.

I feel that marriage so often fails us today not because it no longer has any value for us, but because what we demand of it is too complex and difficult to achieve. It is mostly these expectations which lead to trouble. If we look at it rationally we see that what looks like signs of marriage as we know it coming to an end, are actually signs of adaptation and experiments in survival. What we are seeing is a series of alternatives to conventional marriage. As with all other forms of evolution, we are modifying, rebuilding and redesigning to make it work under present conditions. The conflict we are going through means that it has not changed fast enough to keep up with the changes in our society.

In recent years marriage has been acquiring new meaning and serving, however imperfectly, deep needs we cannot seem to satisfy in any other way. The most important is the need to feel joined in an intimate, exclusive way to another human being. Despite all the talk of troubled male-female relationships, despite all we hear about lack of trust, resentment and anger between men and women, they still want and need each other desperately. They want and need love and even though they may complain and snipe, marriage still provides the environment in which love and security can be engendered.

The more impersonal our world becomes because of increasing technology and change, the more we need an oasis, a small inner world where we can refresh ourselves and renew our strength and energy so that we may go out and face the world with its pressures and worries.

Let's hope that in the nineties we will combine all the lessons we have learned during these years of upheaval and make marriage the satisfying, caring and thoughtful partnership it can be. The potential is still with marriage for a balanced and workable family life and the rewards are worth the perseverance and work required to bring this about. The rest is up to us.

As you would expect, the letters I receive about marriage problems are as individual as the people who write them. Yet they have their similarities too. Most often they are about failed expectations, failure to communicate, money, lack of commitment and caring, romance versus loving, and, always, sex.

Just when I think I have heard them all, I come across a new one, something so unusual or minimal that it is hard to believe it could make waves in a relationship. I am only too aware that it is not always the 'big' problems which create the most havoc. Often it is the day-to-day irritations which are the death of love.

FAILED EXPECTATIONS

Expectations create many of the hurdles in our lives, nowhere more so than in marriage. Mary wrote:

> 'I thought marriage would make me happy, but it
> hasn't. The first few weeks were wonderful, but I don't
> know what's gone wrong. I feel empty and lost. He's
> not the man I thought I married. It was a big mistake.'

Mary is suffering from one of the most common illusions about marriage — that it will fulfil every romantic dream and fantasy and end all feelings of emptiness and frustration. Marriage can and does provide many satisfactions but it is never the perfect solution to personal problems, nor is it a substitute for personal growth and fulfilment or an antidote to loneliness.

Like Mary, many of us marry an idealised character, not a real person with his or her own needs and problems. We set ourselves up for disappointment. Then instead of looking at our own unreasonable projections, we blame the other partner for not fulfilling our fantasy. It is this distorted thinking which leads some people to go from partner to partner in the hope that life will be perfect with the next person, but finding the same unresolved problems in every relationship.

Marriage itself has so many expectations built around it that few people escape *some* disappointment. The following letter from Brian is only one of many on this theme.

> 'My girl and I lived together for three years. Both her parents and mine were divorced and we didn't want the same mess in our lives. But we were so happy together we decided to get married. Well, almost at once everything changed. After only six months of marriage we are talking about divorce.'

I have seen this happen and I am sure it is the back-log of expectations which each partner brings to the relationship which causes the problem. Whereas before you had a lover or companion, now you have a wife or husband with all the role expectations of what a mate should be.

These expectations have been acquired over the years from our parents, our friends, the society we live in and our own observations and conditioning. All these as well as the way we see ourselves, play a powerful role in the way we expect things to be. If each partner is happy with traditional marriage roles, all is well. But today not many couples are content with this stereotype. The only solution is for individuals to work towards their own wholeness by seeing themselves as people first and mates second, and by allowing that right to others as well.

ROMANCE VERSUS LOVE

Over the years I have seen many marriages break down through confusion over the meaning of love. When the intensity of those early years settles into a more companionable love often one, or both partners, begins to feel that love has died, and they try to recapture that 'peak experience' with someone else. What they fail to realise is that the early careless rapture has given way to a lower-key emotion, a deeper kind of loving where tenderness, loyalty, deep attachment and caring play a greater part than passion. This is not to say that the more peaceful kind of love is without its more passionate moments, only that these moments have decreased and changed over the years. Yet some partners are prepared to break up years of shared life together on this hiccup alone. Derek had fallen into that trap:

> 'After six years of marriage I no longer feel the same about my wife as I did when we first married. I'm fond of her and respect her but have no other feelings. We have two children and lately our sex life is almost non-existent. I feel there is no future for us together but don't want to hurt her.'

I wondered how he could say he had no feelings when in the same breath he said he was fond of her, respected her and didn't wish to hurt her. What else is this but real loving, was the question I wanted to put to him. What he was really saying was that he no longer felt the urgent, passionate desire to make love to her. It had not occurred to him that marriage and parenthood take some of the *zing* and fantasy out of sex. Nor had it occurred to him that what he could have in its place was something deeper, more satisfying and exciting — a real, all-round love expressed in a hundred ways including sexually. I suggested that leaving the children with friends or grandparents and having an occasional naughty weekend away was an excellent way to rediscover each other as lovers, rather than always relating as 'mum' or 'dad'. Once the thrill of the chase is gone, it is up to each individual to create the circumstances where it is easy to rediscover each other as lovers, instead of in the humdrum way of daily routine.

This next letter from Joy highlighted one of the most common myths about romance versus love. Unless it is dangerous and exciting and painful, goes the myth, it is only second-rate and not worth having.

> 'I married my husband for security, and because I
> needed someone dependable as my early life had been
> spent going from one relative to another. He has been
> kind, safe and a wonderful provider, but now after ten
> years of marriage and three children, I feel I missed
> out on romance and excitement and long for someone to
> sweep me off my feet. I realise now it was a mistake to
> settle for security.'

The error many women make is to think in terms of *either* security or romance. We all need both, men as well as women, and how can anyone draw a line down the middle and say they married for this or that reason? Obviously Joy married the man she needed and that turned out to be a good choice. It is to her credit that with such an unstable background she intuitively knew what was right for her wellbeing and serenity. And what is romance, anyway, but the attractive outer wrapping of love?

'Instead of whingeing about the lack in your life,' I wrote back, 'why not try introducing a little romance into your husband's? After all, it takes two to tango, as the old song says, and you might be surprised at his reaction.'

I ended my letter with some heartfelt advice: 'Don't jeopardise a good marriage over what is only a fantasy which *you* can bring to life with your husband if you so desire.'

TOTAL TOGETHERNESS CAN STIFLE

Another expectation which creates problems is 'total' togetherness. When it was first touted as the ideal in marriage, it sounded like the recipe for perfect bliss. In reality it demands more than any one person can give without feeling that they are being sucked dry. We all need space even from those we love most if our energies are to flow and not become blocked. If there is no outside input from other people we have nothing fresh and new to bring to each other and our intimate relationship is stifled.

It is only in recent times that we have come to expect our mate to fill our every need and spend every leisure moment with us. In the past, men more often enjoyed the company of fellow club members, sporting associates and friends, while women turned to female relatives for closeness and emotional support.

Today we expect our mate to be our friend, an understanding confidant on whom we can dump all our problems, our companion in fun, our comforter, our nurse when we are ill, our helpmate, an income earner, housekeeper or maintenance person, a loyal pal and a good lover. All this is too much to ask of any person. No wonder many marriages sag under the pressure of so many demands. Togetherness that is balanced encourages intimacy. Total togetherness crowds and stifles and deadens romance. Kahlil Gibran's words: 'Let there be spaces in your togetherness,' is a motto every married couple should heed.

The need for total togetherness seems to bother wives more than husbands and I receive many letters on this topic. Peter wrote about his wife's unrealistic demands:

> 'My job involves a lot of travelling and my wife has never liked this. She says she gets lonely. I've tried very hard to get her interested in hobbies and local activities and have always encouraged her to have friends and expand her own horizons. But nothing seems to work. She wants me to change my job which I'd be crazy to do, especially at this time. She doesn't even seem to be all that interested in our son, aged three. Often when I'm home, she takes him to her mother's so that she and I can be alone. All I want is a happy family life. Can you tell me how to get it?'

'She seems desperate to have you actually by her side to feel secure and happy. Insecurity to this degree is usually a childhood problem and I'm sure she'd like to be rid of it herself and enjoy a relaxed family life when you're there — and a full, happy life when you're not. Was she left alone a lot as a child, or did she fear her parents leaving her? Do all you can to get her to talk things over with a marriage counsellor. Your own happiness depends on sorting out her unhappiness.'

Here is a letter on a similar theme from Sandra:

'We've been happily married for two years and I know
my husband loves me as much as I love him. But now
he wants to change his job for one that will mean he'll
be away for two weeks at a time. He says the extra
money will get us on our feet faster. I'm so upset
because I'm afraid he'll fall for other women when he's
away from me, and I've begged him not to change jobs.
This has made him angry and cold towards me.'

My answer was frank. 'If your husband is an ordinary, good
man who loves you and feels loved by you, then it could have
been a kick in the teeth to discover that you see him as an
unfaithful, weak lecher while he's away. Your pleading probably
makes him feel trapped too. Get back close to him, restore his
self-esteem and freedom of choice, and you can make every
homecoming another honeymoon.'

JEALOUSY — THE GREEN-EYED MONSTER

Jealousy is an emotion which can afflict people of any age. We
don't like to admit to it, but it's there in all of us in varying
degrees. It becomes a real problem when it is allowed to
become all-consuming. The letters concerning jealousy are
nearly always from women but this first one is from Steve and
told me more about Steve and his marriage than he imagined.

'You don't often include letters from men, but I'm
desperate. It's my jealousy. My wife has taken a job in
a club which involves some weekend and evening work.
We have three school-age children, and family life is
going down the drain. What's worse is that my wife
has made a new circle of friends in this job and is
constantly going to parties without me. It makes me
boil with rage, thinking of her mixing with other men.
I've thought of going out on my own too — but she
shows no sign of being jealous about me and in any
case, I haven't any friends. My whole life is centred on

my wife. What can I do to make our marriage as happy
as it used to be before she went to work?'

'I wonder how happy your wife considered the marriage
before she took this job? As I see it, she is behaving like a caged
bird suddenly set free. I feel she is reacting this way because she
feels stifled. On your own admission, you depend on her for all
your social and emotional needs. You're unsure of yourself, and
of being loved and wanted, which is a great burden for any wife
to bear for long. But your jealous rage and your wife's indifference are not the ways to handle a problem. It would help if you
had a bit of a separate life for yourself — not to make her jealous
but to give you more self-confidence, and ease your wife's feelings of being trapped and stifled. All marriages change over the
years and your wife obviously enjoys her independence, but it
doesn't necessarily mean she has tired of you or her family. In
fact, her going to work has probably saved your marriage.'

Jacki wrote:

'My problem is one of jealousy. I don't know how you
can help me but please try. I can't stand my husband
to look at TV ads or at naked women or anything to do
with women. I have four beautiful children by him and
he just can't understand me. I was all right before we
had children but after the first one I began to feel like
this and I'm getting worse. I think my husband is
losing his love for me over this. He always comes
straight home from work, but I'm very depressed.'

'Do you really believe your problem would be solved if you
blindfolded your husband?' I asked. 'Of course it wouldn't, for
the simple reason that all the doubts are in your own mind, and
they are doubts about yourself. What about making a few
changes to break this destructive cycle? Take up any sort of
part-time job outside the home, or join a club or group according
to your interests — tennis, crafts, community work, anything
which allows you to mix with other people. What you are suffering from is a bad case of the miseries. When you feel like that,
everything seems wrong. So get out there and make things

happen. You'll feel more confident and these unhappy feelings will vanish. And how about a weekend away with your husband to restore your faith in each other?'

WE DON'T TALK ANYMORE

Communication is expressed in many ways. It does not mean to agree all the time, as some people think. It can mean talking softly, shouting, arguing. Even saying nothing can be a form of communication. Talking honestly is the best way. Cathy wrote:

> 'My husband is a wonderful guy. He helps me in the
> house, never goes out without me, gives me his wages
> packet every week and each morning when he wakes
> up he tells me he loves me. But he doesn't say
> anything when we make love and I get the feeling he
> doesn't want me but only does it to make me happy.
> Am I expecting too much?'

On one level Cathy is expecting too much. He sounds like a man in a million who shows his love for his wife with every breath he draws. But I feel Cathy is unsure of her own worth. She is not nourished by his expressions of love. It is important not only to give love but also to receive it when it is given and I feel Cathy cannot do this. She needs constant reassurance but the deficit is never filled. Yet she has every right to regard lovemaking as a form of communication in which words, as well as physical closeness, play a part. Words can impart a tenderness which nothing else can do. Her mistake is in assuming that he should know what she wants and give it to her. This inability to express a need creates more misunderstandings than almost any other. There is nothing wrong with asking for what pleases you, for what you want, and Cathy needs to do this. Being honest with him would free her from the irritation and resentment which keeps her focussed on what she is missing, rather than concentrating on the joy they could be experiencing.

This next letter from Hal appeared trivial at first, yet there were many underlying truths in it.

> 'Why are women so greedy for compliments? I say the
> fact that a husband comes home every night, gives her
> his paypacket and doesn't beat her is compliment
> enough! My wife is at me all the time to say 'nice
> things' to her, but I feel a proper fool. All that sweet
> talk is a waste of time.'

It seems that Hal has never stopped to consider that the 'sweet talk' he disparages can make all the difference between a flat, lifeless marriage and one that has some joy in it. I agree that in a good relationship you don't need a lot of words, but all of us, men as well as women, need the occasional compliment, words of praise or appreciation. To Hal, 'nice words' are just that and no more. To women they mean tenderness and romance and encourage a deeper intimacy. Many of Hal's generation were brought up to believe that real men don't 'carry on with all that sweet talk'. It was seen as a weakness.

Perhaps this was the way Hal's parents behaved and that conditioning is hard to change. It is also true that some men find it hard to express their feelings. I think Hal's reluctance to say nice things to his wife reflects an unwillingness to give of himself. What he does not know is that if he gives totally he'll get back totally. I told Hal that no matter how deeply you felt about someone, if you never let them know in words as well as actions, it allows misunderstandings to creep in. And I suggested that he use a bit of humour to break the tension he feels. He could also bring his wife flowers or chocolates or some other little surprise occasionally to let her know he thinks her special. And I said that, as with most things, 'nice talk' gets easier with practice.

Boredom in varying degrees creeps into many marriages and it is caused by and is the cause of many people failing to communicate. In Bill's case it was extreme.

> 'My wife and I have never had children and when we're
> alone at home she watches television in silence or
> sleeps. She refuses to go for a walk with me or even to
> go out for a meal, but amazingly she livens up at once
> if friends drop in or agree to go out with us. There's
> no warmth or excitement between us, and on the rare

occasions we have sex she makes out she's doing me a big favour. She doesn't seem to be bored with life in general, only with me. What can I do to bring back love and a bit of joy and sparkle to our marriage?'

I told him: 'It sticks out a mile that from your wife's point of view, you're simply *not there*. And you can really only be a "non-person" to others in this way if you are, to some extent, lifeless and joyless in yourself. This is not to say you're dull right through — no one is — nor that you have to change your nature. It's asking you to look beyond your chair in front of the television, and other boring habits, to all the other people, places, interests, causes, points of view and enthusiasms to be explored out there. You have to be an *interested* person before you can be an *interesting* one. A lively, love-filled marriage can only come about from the liveliness and loving of the two people in the marriage — nowhere else.'

Helen wrote:

'Soon after I had my baby, my husband started shift work. This means he goes straight to bed just as I'm getting up. And when he gets up in the afternoon he doesn't bother with me and the baby, but just sits and reads. He says he's tired of my whingeing. We don't make love any more, either. What can I do to stop my marriage breaking up?'

'This is a change-over time for both of you,' I said, 'and you need each other's help, so try not to quarrel or complain. I think you'll have to change your routine a little so that some small part of the day, perhaps the late evening before he goes to work, is just for you and him. See if you can save your complaints for someone who'll understand — your mother, or an aunt or a friend. At this stage he's not prepared to understand because all he wants and needs from you is the reassurance that he still comes first in your life. If you change, he'll have to change too.'

'HENPECKED' HUSBANDS

Most of the letters I receive are from women. Men don't admit to their problems so easily, but occasionally they write and then we see the other side of the coin. Here's Bruce's letter:

'I've been married for two years, and quite frankly, I don't wonder marriage is going out of fashion. My wife seems to think I should be constantly at her beck and call. I help her with the housework when needed as she works fulltime, but it's as if she can't bear to see me having a moment to myself. I like reading for instance, but as soon as I sit down, she calls me to lend her a hand. We always watch the TV programs she chooses, go out when and where she decides and she has even taken to telling me when to go to bed. Surely this is not what marriage should be like? I still love her but feel that if things go on like this I will have to leave her. Or do you think I should just put up with it?'

Bruce's solution of 'putting up with it' wouldn't work. Underneath he'd be unhappy and resentful. There couldn't possibly be any love or respect on either side and in the end, it would be as destructive to the marriage for her to do all the taking, as for him to do all the giving.

My advice was, for both their sakes, that he stop giving in so meekly and work out a plan for living together which gives them both time to call their own. I suggested that perhaps she was under pressure because of her two jobs — home and work — and therefore needed more help than if she were not earning. But sharing the chores can still be arranged so that he can have some time off duty.

'As to the decisions about outings, TV, bedtime and so on', I wrote back, 'well, it's up to you to express wishes and stick to them. By having a mind of your own and using it, you become her equal and not her enemy.'

A partnership can only be loving and lasting when it is between two equals. I urged him to see a marriage guidance counsellor with or without his wife. He obviously needed a boost to his self-confidence in order to set things right.

Peter wrote:

> 'How does one cope with a nagging wife? My wife can
> be happy, fun-loving and a joy for weeks on end, then
> she starts nagging me and our teenage children
> unmercifully, and never for any good reason that we
> can make out. If we try to argue back, she either goes
> into a rage or weeps for hours. I'd like to help her if I
> could, but I don't understand what triggers off these
> episodes.'

He sounded sincere and anxious to help, and I tried to enlighten him.

'It's obvious that what she nags about and who she nags are relatively unimportant, so this means that there's something nagging *her* at these times. It could be that she is pre-menstrual, or she may be under some emotional pressure, such as feeling taken-for-granted or left out by the rest of the family.

'Try to bring this up at a moment when she is not tense, and I'm sure she'll be as anxious as you to find the real cause of her outbursts. If it is pre-menstrual tension, her doctor can help. If it's to do with feelings between you, or in the family, then you can work to remove the source of resentment. Even just bringing it out into the open and having you acknowledge how she feels, may resolve the problem.'

CHARITY BEGINS AT HOME — DOESN'T IT?

The next two letters show how even unselfish behaviour can create problems in some cases.

Pam wrote:

> 'My husband can't say no to anyone, and I feel very
> neglected because of other people's demands on his
> time. Our home is open house to all his family and
> friends and he's always rushing around fixing things,
> doing things for other people. He lends anything and

everything we've got. I know he loves me, but I feel so
hurt and fed up. What can I do to make him wake up
to himself?'

'Frankly, I don't think you should try,' I replied. 'It would be
far better if you could learn to share him. Love's not rationed,
you know, and it isn't true that the more he gives to others, the
less there'll be for you. In fact, the more love he has to spread
around, the bigger your share of it. Accept him as he is and join
him in spirit, even if it is not practical for you to be quite as
open-handed as he is. Now and again it would do you good to
imagine having a husband at the other extreme, mean with
everything, his possessions, his time, his help and his love. That
would really make you a neglected wife.'

Andrew wrote:

'I do voluntary work locally in the evenings and at
weekends. It's mainly with the elderly, and my
children, who are in their early teens, are starting to
join in. But my wife resents this and is forever
reminding me that charity begins at home. As I have
no intention of giving up this community help, can you
suggest any way I can make my wife happier about it?'

'You don't have to give up your community help,' I wrote, 'but
make certain you're being as charitable as you can be to your
wife's needs as an individual. This means trying to understand
what bugs her about your out-of-the-home activities. Does she
feel left out? Do you have time to talk together sometimes on an
intimate level, just you and her? Does she feel neglected or
lonely? What satisfactions does she have to match those you get
from voluntary work? Can you help her find some?

'While I applaud and admire your attitude which is also a great
example for your children, I must advise you not to let the
elderly monopolise all your caring instincts — there is a happy
medium, so try to find it.'

SHARING THE LOAD — MONEY PROBLEMS

I am sure many young mothers can identify with Lucy's problem — I know it brought back many memories for me of those early years of marriage and motherhood!

> 'We have a baby son and are very happy. My husband is
> kind but we just can't afford nice clothes for me or
> expensive make-up and I often feel very shabby. I feel
> selfish and guilty wanting things I can't have,
> especially as my husband works so hard and does
> without things and never complains. But I can't stop
> these thoughts from coming into my head.'

'It's not wrong or selfish to long for something — we all do it so there's no need to feel guilty,' I wrote back. 'When other needs come first, like providing for the home and a baby, then you put aside this natural wish for lovely clothes and expensive make-up and do the best with what you've got. In the meantime, there's no need to look shabby — and I'm sure you only *think* you look shabby. I know many young mothers who buy inexpensive clothes and add their own individual touches with scarves, belts and costume jewellery and end up looking stunning. Some have told me they shop at opportunity stores and always manage to look good.

'And why not learn to sew. That is always a great help in making you look well-dressed on a very limited budget. And you don't need the most expensive make-up to look good. Your youth and freshness are beauty enough with very little help.'

One thing that many married people argue over is money. Here is Chloe's letter:

> 'Ever since we were married three years ago, the only
> rows my husband and I have had are about money and
> his management of it. He admits he's always been
> afraid of financial commitment and says he can't
> explain why he is so hopeless at looking after this side
> of things. I've always managed rather well with savings

and money matters but I can't convince him that he'd
be just as competent if he tried. He's level-headed and
loves me very much and I love him, so how do we cope
with this?'

Chloe does not see that the solution is easier than she imagines. She should take over the money management in the family — lots of wives do. And an increasing number of husbands daunted by domestic responsibilities on top of their work pressures are happy about this. It is no use sticking rigidly to the old idea that the man took care of money matters. Many things have changed and this is one of them. It's all a matter of aptitudes of who does what. There was a time not so long ago when no man worthy of his name would change a baby's nappy, yet now I see young fathers who are wonderfully apt at looking after their babies.

But I would urge Chloe not to take over the family finances as a matter of her competence and his incompetence. It's simply a matter of sharing the load, so that each tackles the area of responsibility he/she feels confident about. Undoubtedly there are things he manages better than Chloe. By each doing what they do best, there is an increase in confidence and involvement which adds strength individually and as a team.

The next letter is more complex and touches on more than money problems. Margot writes:

'Although we have been married fifteen years, I have
never known what my husband earns. I have always
managed to run the house on what he has given me,
but now I'm fighting a losing battle. The price of food
has gone up so much that I just can't make ends meet.
My husband likes good meals — no making do for him
— but he refuses to believe that money is not elastic.
How can I make him see that he is being unfair?'

Marriage is a partnership and both partners have every right to know what money they have or haven't got. Even in these so-called enlightened times, too many women are kept in the dark about family finances by being handed a sum of money and told to make do. If I were Margot, I'd keep a list of every item purchased, together with all available receipts and price labels. She should show them to her husband and let him see what she does with her budget. If he remains stubborn, I'd simply make cheaper meals, still keeping records and receipts. When he complains she should tell him to make do or raise the allowance. And if she thinks he can do better, let him try! A stint of shopping brings many men to their senses.

Jean's letter was one of many I receive these days on the subject of working wives.

'In the middle of 1989 I went back to work as a secretary, because we couldn't manage on my husband's salary and save for our home as well. I am well-paid although I don't earn as much as my husband, but already, after a little over a year, our marriage of two and a half years is breaking up because we can't work out how my salary is to be used. My husband expects me to take out money for fares and lunch and then put all the rest into a household account. I want a little independence and although I am prepared to help out by pulling with him in building our future, I don't intend to give up everything and have to ask him every time I need a new pair of pantyhose. What are your views on this? I don't want our marriage to break up.'

I wrote back: 'With so many women back in the workforce nowadays, letters such as yours are more frequent in my mail. Money seems such a sad reason for a marriage to break up. After all, working towards something, whether it's a house or a trip or simply to keep financially afloat, should bring a couple closer together. Often though, the problem goes deeper than mere cash. Some husbands feel inadequate when their wife goes out to work, and while welcoming the help, feel that their pride and self-confidence have been shaken and undermined. From a practical point of view, I'd suggest that you both contribute what you consider a fair proportion of your salaries to a joint account from which all household expenses will be met, including the amount to be put aside for your future home. What is left over from that, you can each keep for personal expenditure. If things don't improve, a session or two with a marriage guidance counsellor would help.'

AN EQUAL PARTNERSHIP

I receive many letters from women who complain that their husbands are never willing to help them with jobs around the house. The greatest number of these letters are from pregnant women. Joy wrote:

'I know my husband loves me and he really is very thoughtful in most ways, especially now I'm expecting our first baby. But he always gets irritated when I ask him to help me with jobs that need doing around the house at weekends or in the evenings. He makes the excuse that he was just about to do something else. I'm getting the nursery ready and some of the jobs are too much for me and I don't understand why he won't help. It's not that he actually refuses — he just says: "All right, I'll do it later", or "What's the hurry? I'll do it tomorrow". I hate to keep on asking. It makes me feel he doesn't care.'

I replied: 'Most husbands would, I'm sure, help out a lot more if their wives used better tactics in enlisting help, and that's where the problem is. Like many women — especially when they're pregnant — you're inclined to see his willingness to help as something to do with how much he cares for you, rather than a simple matter of convenience. That makes it all an emotional matter instead of a practical one, which in turn makes you hammer away irrationally at getting him to prove he cares, instead of rationally making it easier for him to help. It's likely, you see, that he has his time at home roughly mapped out, so that unexpected requests for help can be quite maddening. Why don't you plan ahead too, and give him advance notice of when you'll need his help with a particular chore? It's really just a matter of timing.'

LACK OF COMMITMENT AND CARING

Over the years I have always advised trying every possible solution before giving up on a marriage. But I have learned that where there is no commitment or caring, the relationship is doomed. Marcia's marriage was such a one.

'Although we are living under the same roof, my husband and I separated a month ago after only two and a half years of marriage. He is hot-tempered, foul-mouthed and quite spoilt, but I love him. From the time we married he expected me to take the place of his mother but would never recognise my needs. He says nobody needs to talk about problems or be shown love. I go to marriage guidance but he refuses to go. I am 21, he is 26. Our son is two and needs a father — I missed not having one around very much. He says the marriage is finished unless I cook, clean and shut up.'

I felt she had made a bad choice and her only solution was to cut her losses and try again, but clearly this was not what she wanted to hear. My intuition told me that having grown up without a father she did not have a very good idea of what a caring man should be. Her lack during childhood of a model had no doubt influenced her choice of husband. This man's idea that you don't discuss problems or show love indicates a repressed person who has not had enough mothering and has built walls around his emotions for fear of being hurt. He has been brought up to consider no one except himself and I see no possibility of change. Some people are married to themselves and should never marry anyone else. He was one of these men. Marcia is trying to hold the marriage together by going to marriage guidance and this is not necessarily wasted. It will give her new insights into her own behaviour which will give her a broader view and a greater range of choices. But she can't do it all no matter how well-intentioned. I urged her not to try another relationship while in this vulnerable state but to wait until she has sorted out her feelings. Otherwise she will repeat the same mistake.

My first reaction to Barbara's letter was 'Why does she stay?'

> 'We've been married for nine years and have no
> children. My husband never takes me anywhere, has
> never taken me on a holiday and never allowed me to
> have friends over. Pleading with him does no good, it
> just makes him angrier than usual. Since I cannot
> force him to treat me like an equal, how do I get a life
> of my own? I had to give up my job three years ago
> because of a long illness and although I am fully
> recovered now, I haven't tried for another position.'

There is no joy, no caring or affection here. He sounds like a man who thinks he is always right and who will not change his views for anyone. Of course, Barbara has played along with his game. No doubt her self-image and self-esteem were so low she did not think she deserved any better. I made an educated guess that her long illness was her body's response to a situation that was making her desperately unhappy. The only hope I see for her is that her new found awareness will impel her to get out of this prison. But I see no hope that this marriage will survive.

Her first step should be to do what she needs to do regardless of his wishes and certainly without waiting for permission. She could look for a job if that is what she wants, join a club or two according to her interests and meet friends at their home or hers. She might even consider leaving him if that is the only way to freedom. Perhaps the thought of losing her could shake him out of his tyrannical role. Sometimes such tyrants in the home are like school bullies who cave in when their power is challenged by someone who is not afraid. I urged Barbara to have marriage guidance counselling if she felt it would give her the back-up to stand up to him. As things are she has nothing to lose. But she must follow through to bring about the change she wants. Freedom is there for *us* to take. No one will hand it to us.

Judy's letter talked about a marriage that was not a marriage at all. The image it conjured up for me was of two dumb animals yoked together and following a rut which was getting deeper and deeper.

> 'I am getting tired of living with my husband. I don't
> know whether it is his fault or mine, but now, in our

forties, we are drifting further and further apart. I
really don't know how he feels about our life together
because I can't talk about it, but to me it just seems to
have been a big waste of time. We have worked in the
same jobs in the same places all the time and all our
friends are working colleagues. Our lives are so dull
and I'm so unhappy.'

This is a clear picture of two people who are held together in misery and nothing else. There is no caring, no shared feelings of hope for the future. I felt they had probably followed the crowd and drifted into marriage. They had no expectations and put in no effort. I imagined they started off with good intentions but their marriage shows what happens when a relationship is neglected like an abandoned garden — the weeds take over.

Judy's admission that she can't talk to him about how she feels is a problem I hear so often. And yet how can such an intimate relationship as marriage blossom and grow if nothing is ever brought out into the open and discussed? It's as if people are afraid that if they speak the truth the union can't survive.

The opposite is true. It is this tacit agreement not to make waves which kills whatever chance two people have of making a relationship work. If there is a recipe for disaster, this is it. In silence each assumes that the other knows what he or she is thinking, but nothing is ever said. That is how misunderstandings occur, how feelings are hurt sometimes beyond forgiveness.

If only people were more honest and open, I am certain half the problems I read about would never happen.

INAPPROPRIATE BEHAVIOUR

Mavis wrote about a problem which crops up now and again, but, thankfully, not too often.

'My husband's 52 and I'm 54. I don't know whether it's
his age, but he's grown very silly about young girls. He
loves their company and plays up to them in a way
which makes me feel physically ill. He never says a
kind word to me any more. I've spent hours crying over
his unkind behaviour.'

'Well, dry your tears, put aside the misery and stop resisting your husband's behaviour,' I replied. 'Don't you know that what we resist is what we get? The point is that you are both at an age when you to need reassurance about still being attractive and lovable. He gets *his* reassurance because young girls respond to him. You make no attempt to get reassurance, but resent the fact that your husband *is* bothering.

'The whole point is that you could both be getting what you need from each other. Make him feel he's an attractive person who matters to you and he'll make you feel the same. He might still fuss a bit over girls, but it won't upset you nearly as much as it does now. If you can look at his antics with a certain detachment — even seeing the funny side — you'll be amazed at how trivial the whole problem becomes, and how much wind you'll take out of his sails.'

IS HE RIGHT FOR MY DAUGHTER?

Nora's letter expressed concern for her daughter's engagement to a man of 50. I felt her fears were unfounded, and told her so.

'My only daughter is engaged to a man of nearly 50 who still lives with his mother, a widow. My daughter's 35 and this is her first romance. She has never been so happy, and I like the man, but I can't help feeling very anxious about the marriage. Can a man who has avoided marriage for so long, and is bound to be set in his ways, ever make a good husband?'

'Your doubts are understandable,' I replied, 'but it is pointless talking of 'a good husband' as if there were a model type with certain characteristics including, it seems, a willingness to try marriage early in life, regardless of whether this suits his nature and circumstances. Your daughter is evidently not one to play the field, nor is he. Both may have been waiting for a like-minded partner and both may be quite capable of adapting to marriage, late as it is. So stop worrying and be happy for them.'

PHYSICAL AND EMOTIONAL ABUSE

There are always two or three letters regarding domestic violence in my mail, most of them from women who are on the receiving end. This next letter was from a man who resorted to violence to his regret.

> 'My wife and I have been married for six years and have a daughter aged five. About a month ago I did a silly thing — I lost my temper and hit my wife. I hit her once before and have regretted it ever since. This time my wife walked out on me and our little girl. She says she is not coming back because she's afraid of me. I have begged her to forgive me and pleaded with her to think it over. I love her and am deeply sorry for what I did. How can I convince her that I have changed my ways?'

I told him that I didn't blame his wife for reacting as she did to his violence especially as it wasn't the first time.

'You say you regretted it,' I wrote back, 'but it didn't stop you from repeating it, did it? So how can she be sure you won't hit her again?'

I assured him that the only way he could convince her he wanted to change was to discuss his feelings and underlying aggression in an intelligent and sensible way. 'Professional counselling is what you need,' I wrote. 'Make an appointment with a counsellor at Family Life or Centacare and ask your wife to come with you.'

Some months later I received a letter from Jill, his wife, in which she said that counselling had put them on the road to better understanding and their marriage was more satisfying and peaceful than in the past.

Lack of caring can be expressed in many ways — passively, as in the failure to acknowledge the other's needs, or aggressively, by not recognising how abuse can damage a relationship.

In this next letter, from Susan, we see how emotional abuse can be as damaging as physical abuse, but in a different way.

'I am writing this letter in desperation. I feel I will go crazy trying to socialise the man I have been living with for the last two years. He is eight years younger than me. I work as a dress designer and Jack works in a factory but constantly job hops. If I bring my problems home to discuss, I am told he doesn't want to ruin his day by listening to my problems. If he knows I have spent a lot of time preparing a special meal he will say "No thank you, I'll get something later". If I bring home a gift or a special treat he says "Don't do me any favours, I don't need them". He will suggest an outing but if I look as if I'm getting excited about it he will decide not to go. If I have some exciting news for him or if I look as if I am happy, he will knock the polish off it straight away with something really cutting. He enrolled in a course and I encouraged him, so he dropped out. If the cat comes near me or my daughter Gina (she is five years old and not his daughter), he makes some unpleasant remark under his breath. He constantly talks non-stop about himself and things he has done, which are just fantasies. He overtalks you if you try to comment. If I ask about his day, I am interfering in his life. If we have visitors he shuts himself in his room. Another strange thing is that if I raise my hand quickly for any reason, he flinches as if I were going to hit him. He tells me he loves me but how can I believe him? He is very good-looking and I am so attracted to him I can't leave him. I'm so unhappy. Can you help me?'

What came across in this letter was a man who had been so damaged in his early years he could only relate to women by punishing them in a sadistic way. I asked myself 'Why does she stay?' but could find no answer. People are drawn together for a variety of reasons, some of them apparently inexplicable. I surmised that he must have *some* good qualities which filled her needs some of the time. It was clear to me that what he felt for her was not love, but a dependent need. That she stayed despite his treatment of her showed that she was needy in her own way.

In fact, they were both locked into each other's destructive behaviour patterns. He needed professional intensive therapy and even then there was no guarantee that he would change. She was in a catch-22 situation — if she tried to placate him he reacted viciously, if she stood up to him he was worse. Her options were limited and I advised her to get out of the relationship before she herself was destroyed. I have seen many such cases where women have been driven to nervous breakdowns and even suicide from 'trying to make it right' for men who were determined to make them wrong.

Jack sounded like a man with appallingly low self-esteem and a totally unrealistic idea of himself. The clue here was his need to make up stories about himself and his achievements. We all tell the occasional white lie. It becomes destructive when we believe our own lies. Jack feels he is so worthless he needs to believe his fantasies. He is always in conflict at work and with friends because people don't relate to him in the way he sees himself, so he blames others when things don't work out.

Susan's mistake is that she is trying to communicate on a rational, realistic level but Jack's world is not rational or sane. He has been so damaged, the slightest word or action triggers off his punishing mode so that he is not even aware he is doing it. I wondered if Jack was not more seriously disturbed emotionally and mentally than appeared at first. I hoped the counsellor he might have gone to see would pick up the signs and refer him to a psychiatrist. I sensed that he had been physically abused as well as emotionally harmed (the fact that he flinches if someone raises their arm is a clear indication of fear).

I felt Jack's relationship with his mother was probably the basis of his inability to relate to women. Men like Jack could never please their mother; whatever he did it was never enough. The tragedy is that men who grow up with this sort of deprivation learn to play the part of 'poor thing' in order to encourage women to help them and like them. But once a woman begins to care about him she becomes vulnerable, which puts him in a powerful position and then he can't contain the deep-rooted hate and resentment he felt for his mother for not giving him the love he wanted. In this confusion of feelings, the wife or girl-friend becomes the mother and he punishes her as such. What-ever had happened in his childhood, he was now punishing every woman he met as though she was his mother.

There are many men like Jack and they are always without insight and compassion. The only way they feel 'powerful' is to cut someone down and they do it without compunction. It's the only time they feel potent. What Susan didn't know at this stage was that by being forgiving and allowing herself to be treated like this she was deepening and strengthening Jack's warped belief system. Jack needed intensive therapy.

As far as Susan was concerned I felt she was emotionally needy and too afraid to take risks where relationships were concerned. She lacked confidence in herself and in her ability to hold a man. It was likely that her father (the first man in her life) had not been a good role model of what a caring man should be and she still did not know. I also suggested that Susan have counselling for her own benefit. Otherwise she would go on attracting men who mistreated her in this way.

AND, ALWAYS, SEX

A great number of letters are related to sex, either too much or too little or not good enough. Such was Joan's letter:

> 'This letter is difficult to write but you are my last
> hope. My husband is 43, I am 40 and we have been
> married 18 years, happily, I might add. My husband
> has always seemed satisfied with our love life, but in
> the past few months he has changed so much I don't
> know what to think. He has become so demanding and
> passionate and keeps at me to try new ways of making
> love. I feel we are getting a bit old for this sort of
> thing, but I'm afraid he might turn to some other
> woman, so I try to please him. Do you think I should
> discourage his behaviour or should I accept it?'

Many of the women who write to me would say Joan doesn't know just how lucky she is to have a husband who still wants her passionately after so many years of marriage. My advice to her was not to 'accept' his attentions, but to welcome them with open arms, literally! I can't tell for certain why he has suddenly developed the exotic tastes Joan hints at — perhaps he has heard that when a man reaches middle age it's time for him to liven up his sex life while he is still capable of enjoying it. Or maybe he has read an article which has given him new insights into what erotic delights he has been missing by being dull. But why should the reason matter? What does matter is Joan's attitude to all this. To tell the truth, she sounds more astonished than put off. I have a feeling that secretly she rather enjoys this new-style sex. 'So why not shed those old guilty feelings,' I wrote to her, 'and enjoy the fun?' But I also added that her husband should have a medical check-up. Middle-aged men with prostate problems sometimes show a sudden and overwhelming increase in libido.

I receive a lot of letters about the following problem:

'I am 28, have been married for eight years and have a two-year-old child. My problem is that my husband and I have not had sex at all since the conception of the child. We have always had an irregular sex pattern, making love once monthly or every few months with me always making the first advance. Our lovemaking is always over in a few minutes and I was never satisfied or aroused because of this. My husband witnessed our child's birth which was very painful. Could this be holding him back in case I got pregnant again? I often feel that he looks on me as a mother figure now rather than as a wife and lover. I have encouraged and reassured him that it's okay to make love now but he always has some excuse. I would be happy with just some caressing and petting, but no go. He loves me dearly, I know, but I'm wondering if I love him any more. He is 31 and in excellent health. I'm desperate for advice, as I don't know where to turn.'

It is clear from this letter that Anne's husband has always had a low sex-drive and that he suffers from premature ejaculation. No doubt he has unresolved conflicts with his mother and has a

great fear of inadequacy which was probably exacerbated by
Anne taking the lead. I also feel that he was not emotionally
ready for fatherhood or to witness the birth of his child. Too
many of his own hang-ups are getting in the way. In many cases,
impairment of sexual function originates from feelings of fear,
guilt and anger. Another possible explanation is that of *transfer-
ence*, which means that he is experiencing his wife as someone
else. His attitude towards his mother is being transferred to his
wife, and so sex becomes impossible.

All this is at a subconscious level, of course, but nothing can
be done until he recognises and deals with it in therapy. The
effect of our birth experience on our lives is being more and
more accepted by therapists. In witnessing the birth of his own
child, Anne's husband was probably shaken by feelings he could
not understand and which came from his own birth experience.
My advice to Anne was to go to Family Planning and ask to be
referred to ASSERT (Australian Society of Sex Educators,
Researchers and Therapists) with her husband. Their problem
could only be overcome if the two people concerned were prepared to work at it together.

Claire's problem is more common than people imagine:

> 'We've been married ten months and I've never had an
> orgasm. I pretend I have so that my husband will
> believe he pleases me. But lately he has been asking me
> more and more if he really satisfies me, and now I'm
> all mixed up and worried about it.'

What Claire does not know is that complete harmony and
satisfaction takes time — sometimes years — but since the journey's so delightful, it's self-defeating to rush up a side street on
your own, which is what she is doing. Pretending is helpful
when established harmony breaks down or when a man badly
needs this kind of reassurance. But in her case it sets up a
phoney basis for their intimate life together, and her husband is
sensing this and is trying to get the truth from her. 'So stress the
pleasure he gives you,' I wrote, 'but be frank about it not being
complete yet and then find the way together.' Reading a couple of
pertinent books would be helpful. *The Joy of Sex* by Alex Comfort is excellent and so is *Becoming Orgasmic — A Sexual*

Growth Programme for Women, by Julia Heiman and L. and J. Lo Piccolo. This latter is available through all University Co-op Bookshops. Another book which I would highly recommend is *Man, Woman and Sexual Desire* by Warwick Williams.

DE FACTO RELATIONSHIPS

It is appropriate here to include one of the new-style marriages we mentioned earlier. Couples living together in a one-to-one relationship which has all the qualities of marriage except for the formalised ceremony, is one of the ways in which marriage is evolving and changing today. The term to describe such a relationship — de facto — has become part of the English language.

Problems arise when one partner, usually the woman, decides that the time has come for them to marry or part. Letters expressing this problem are always tricky to answer. Blackmailing a partner by threatening to leave or even day-to-day harping on marriage are often used as levers to convince the unwilling one that marriage is the only alternative. This approach never works. Resentment at being manipulated undermines the relationship and blame and bitterness for what one partner sees as entrapment destroys all that was good between the two people. I have seen many excellent relationships which had lasted for years break down a few weeks after a wedding which only one of them wanted. Whereas before they had a 'marriage' in everything but the legal sense of the word, they now had a wedding to prove it but no marriage. This letter is a touching example of what I mean.

'For the past ten months I have been in a serious relationship with a wonderful man who loves me dearly and shows it by his actions. I feel totally secure with Mark and love him so much my heart actually aches. We have known each other for eleven years and have been good friends in that time although we were married to other people. Since then I have been widowed and he, divorced. For the past six months we have been living together and our relationship is deepening all the time. My children adore him and call him "Dad" and we are making plans for the future.

The only problem is that I want to make a full
commitment and get married in a year or so, and he is
quite happy to keep things as they are. This makes me
unhappy, as I think marriage is important and I want
my three young children to grow up with that
knowledge. My boyfriend thinks marriage is a farce and
says it doesn't prove your love. I agree with the latter,
but have old-fashioned values and don't feel comfortable
in a de facto relationship. This makes me resentful. I
still love him but my choices seem to be either to live
with him and live with it, or end our beautiful
relationship. We have discussed my feelings and he
hasn't changed his mind. I don't want to force him
into marriage so what should I do? I don't want to end
it as I love him too much, but I don't want resentment
to affect our relationship.'

It seemed to me that both Rebecca and Mark agreed on what
love is, but their assumptions on marriage differed widely and
were getting in the way. Mark was threatened by it, perhaps
because of his previous marriage and it was clear that for
Rebecca, convention was more important than her deepest feelings and intuition. She had probably been brought up in a
strongly conventional environment and would compromise her
own happiness rather than appear to be breaking the rules. Yet
she does not come across as a rigid person. All she needed were
some different points of view to give her another perspective.

In Australia today, the majority of people still choose marriage, but many live in de facto relationships, claiming that a
formalised ceremony does not add to their loving. There are
always many reasons for choosing this path, not all of them
sincere. For some people it is a way of avoiding commitment but
I did not think this was the case with Rebecca and Mark.

'Surely you have more caring and real love in your relationship
than many couples who have a formalised union', I wrote back. I
reminded her that marriage is more for society's convenience
and peace of mind than for the happiness of those concerned. I
said that at this stage of her life companionship was the important thing, and she had it. Rebecca sounded mature and sincere,

and her letter was an authentic expression of her real feelings, and of the knowledge that this was the right relationship for her. Why throw it away so lightly?

My suggestion was that she and Mark should negotiate and set a date in the future for a time to review their ideas about marriage. In the meantime, she could tell the children that she was living in a de facto relationship because of negotiations with her partner. She could admit that it was not the ideal but that the ideal was not possible at this time. I could see that Mark feared being trapped, perhaps because of his first marriage or even earlier experiences. 'If he is to feel safe about marriage,' I wrote back, 'he must see his relationship with you as totally safe and in no way the same as his first marriage.'

I urged Rebecca to allow the relationship to develop at its own rate and told her it would be a mistake to keep talking about marriage. He would see it as pressure to do what he was not ready to do. If he did decide on marriage, he would have to come to that conclusion on his own and not through any coercion on her part.

'Try both of you, not to be too rigid in your thinking,' I wrote. 'It will help you greatly to work this out with the help of a counsellor, either at Family Life or Centacare, or your community health centre. When you talk about it, don't let unnecessary "shoulds" come between your real loving.'

3

Being a Parent

MOST PEOPLE LOVE their children and want what is best for them. And most children love their parents, so why is it that these relationships create so much drama and conflict? Family relationships are all about anger and fear and tears, as well as laughter and loving, and where such intense, basic emotions are involved, it is no wonder problems arise.

Parenting is the most important and potentially rewarding job in the world — and the one for which there is absolutely no training. All people start their lives as parents with natural instincts as to what they should do and end up playing it mostly by ear.

In the past, people learned how to parent from the way they were parented. If they were raised in an atmosphere of love and kindness, they in turn treated their children in the same way. If harsh treatment was their lot, that was the kind of parenting they learned to pass on. The same ideas and precepts were handed down from generation to generation and you didn't even question that you would do as good a job of it as your parents had done.

When I began my column, the family was still regarded as the heartbeat of society. Most of the letters I received told of the usual conflicts between husband and wife, parents and children, lack of communication and uneasy relationships.

Suddenly the sexual revolution was upon us and a lot of parents in their thirties and forties followed their teenagers' lead and began to behave with as much as or more abandon than their children. It was as if they wanted to make up for their own restricted adolescence, and make up for it they did. The changes in society were so tremendous and came at such a fast rate, there was no safe bridge between the two generations. This led to what became a catch phrase — the generation gap. I sat on many a discussion panel of that time and took part in the endless debate. I couldn't see what the fuss was about. A 'gap' between each generation has always existed, but because we had had one hundred years' worth of change in just a few years, the gap seemed to be a lot wider. Parents became anxious and asked a lot of questions.

This was a time when experts and so-called experts were proposing new methods of child-rearing. This would have been a positive step if we had held on to what was of value from the past. Instead it resulted in the abandonment of many instinctual responses and traditions with nothing to replace them. No wonder the basic confidence in child-rearing of past times was undermined. While the new methods made us more aware of some children's needs which had gone unnoticed for so long, they also opened up a Pandora's box of doubt and guilt.

I received a lot of letters especially from mothers in that period, wanting to know more about the 'new child psychology'. They lapped up all that was written about it in books and magazines and wanted yet another opinion — mine. They often misinterpreted what they read and heard, and discipline of any sort was discarded as being harmful to a child's psyche and incompatible with love. Today we are reaping the results of that period of misguided thought. In these past years I have counselled young adults who have admitted to me that growing up with no discipline gave them a feeling of total insecurity.

Another popular fad of that time was the idea that parents were to be their children's friends, rather than mum or dad. While I applaud friendship between parents and children, here was a different concept. All too often parents used it as an excuse to stop being responsible and regress to their youth. I remember receiving letters from confused youngsters who complained of the parents' childish dress and behaviour.

The early eighties saw a gradual change. Preoccupation with sex eased off a little and gave way to preoccupation with the self and material possessions. The favourite expressions of that era were: 'If it feels good, do it,' and 'It's *their* problem, not mine'. Both were cop-outs from taking responsibility for our actions. This became known, understandably, as the 'me' generation.

On the positive side there was an awakened interest in self-development and what motivates and shapes us. People began to question the effect of materialism on our lives and to choose other paths to happiness and fulfilment.

Today, hard times have made us all reassess our values and ambitions. It is heartening to see a return to the more valuable aspects of caring as opposed to clinical parenting, with the addition of modern knowledge and enlightenment. Parents are becoming confident again in the most important job they will ever be called on to do, with far-reaching effect. The next generation — and the next — are bound to reflect this loving confidence. There's hope for us yet!

Each of the letters in this chapter illustrates some aspect of this most basic of all relationships.

PARENTS AS MODELS

The first letter in this section is from Isobel, written in 1985. It echoed what many women were saying at that time.

> 'It's hard being a parent today. You read so many
> conflicting statements about the way to bring up
> children that I am confused and shaky. I always
> thought loving your child was enough.'

I replied, 'Yes, love and understanding are vital in bringing up our children. But after that the most important thing we can do for them is to believe in ourselves as a person and a parent. Parents are the models, the prototypes if you like, from which they learn. If *we* can't cope with life, if we're uncertain, confused and pessimistic, what hope is there for them?

'The fact is, they absorb our values and ideas through their pores as it were, from what we do, from the way we are and not from what we tell them to do. We owe it to them as well as ourselves to be as fulfilled as we can be. It is both exciting and sobering to know that our very best — and our very worst qualities — can be perpetuated in the next generation and in many generations to come.'

TOO MUCH VIOLENCE

Julie's problem is one shared by many concerned parents:

'I am worried by the high content of violence in books, films and television. The general consensus is that it is harmful and should be curbed, but how can you explain its popularity in the community? People queue up to see a violent movie and TV shows filled with blood and gore have the highest ratings, while books with a similar content are best-sellers. Are we becoming callous, or do we use this kind of violence as a sort of catharsis for our own aggression? I have three children and I fear for the future. What do you think?'

'We are living in an age when despite all the talk about communication, awareness and self-fulfilment, a great many people feel bored, ineffectual, alone and empty. In other words, they have lost their capacity to feel, and in a desperate attempt to overcome this, they must search for more and more stimulation. The greater their inner deadness, the greater the violence and 'shock' required to feel anything.

'You are correct in assuming that violence is a form of catharsis for these people. Unfortunately, the stimulation — and 'relief' — derived from violence is never enough to effect a permanent 'cure', and in many cases, such violence can be justly blamed for promoting further violence as disturbed people seek to emulate what they see or read.

'The only way we can get in touch with our feelings and therefore our humanity, is by involvement with our fellow human beings on a meaningful level.'

HIGH EXPECTATIONS

With competition for places in universities and jobs, many parents are placing even more pressure on their children than in the past — often with dire results. Here is John's letter:

'My parents watch over my progress at school like hawks. They want me to be top at everything and

insist that I always choose the highest, and therefore
the hardest, levels of all subjects. I feel so desperate
and jumpy all the time, knowing I don't do nearly as
well as they expect. Now, I'm dreading how they will
react when I fail. They don't seem to be interested in
me, only in how well I can do.'

'You might have it in you to do very well,' I replied, 'but your
parents need to be shown that their attitude is not the way to
support you. I suggest you have a talk to your teacher. Try to draw
your parents into staff-parent meetings or other occasions where
they can meet your teachers and other parents. If their ambitions
are out of line with your capabilities, they should find out now,
rather than expose you to the unfair label of failure.'

MUM'S FAVOURITE

This next letter from Nell throws some light on a frequent problem — mother's favouritism of one child over the others. This
can happen at any age, more especially in the young, but age
does not make it any easier to bear. Here is Nell's letter:

'I come from a big family and since I was a child, I
noticed that my mother favours my youngest sister.
Now we are all grown up and married with children
and it is still happening. If I ask for something or the
others do, the answer is "no". But as soon as my sister
asks they do everything for her. Whatever she does is
great. Even her children are favoured more than all the
other grandchildren. I've had enough of this and feel
like blowing up and telling my mum and sister where
to go. My husband got a job promotion and we are
moving interstate. I'm glad that I can be as far away as
possible from this unfairness around me. I'd like to tell
my mum how I feel but I don't want to hurt her.'

'As long as you are sure the problem does not stem from your
own feelings of jealousy, your mother needs to be told what she
is doing,' I answered. 'People who behave as she does are following their preferences and do not know they are being unfair

until someone draws their attention to it. You don't have to be nasty or make a bad friend of her. Tell her in a calm, considered way how hurt you and your children and the rest of your family are by her obvious favouritism. Since she is probably not aware of it, this may come as a shock to her, but if you say it honestly and openly and without blaming or trying to put her down, it is then up to her how she takes it. She may be a bit toey for a day or two, but it will do her good to know how much she is hurting her family. And by telling her how you feel, you will have removed a lot of the sting that keeps hurting you.'

LEAVING THE CHILDREN AT HOME

Tricia wrote:

'Occasionally my husband and I leave our three children, aged five, seven and nine, with my parents while we go away for a weekend. Friends have told us that this is harmful for the children as they will feel we are rejecting them. Is this possible? We often go on holidays as a family, but also enjoy the break when it's just the two of us. Is this wrong?'

I could reassure her wholeheartedly. 'As long as the children are happy with your parents, it does you all a power of good to part company occasionally. The kids get a break from parental authority, the grandparents can indulge them to their hearts' content, and the parents can relate to each other as lovers, exclusive of family responsibility — a great prescription for everybody.

'I bet your friends wish they had someone to leave their children with for a weekend away! Don't let their remarks spoil what seems a perfect arrangement.'

THE BIOLOGICAL TIME CLOCK

A problem of recent times which my generation did not encounter is the need to have a child and the fear that time is running out. More and more women are writing to me about this. Amanda wrote this letter:

> 'I am an attractive, independent woman of 35 who does
> not have a long-term relationship with a man. I have
> an excellent job with a good salary and can look after
> myself, but lately the desire to be a mother almost
> overwhelms me. I realise time is running out and I am
> now considering having a baby with a man I have been
> going out with since Easter. Would it be better to tell
> him beforehand or to 'play dumb' and become pregnant
> without him knowing? I am sure there are pros and
> cons to my argument, so can you please help me make
> up my mind whether to go ahead or forget it?'

I felt that what Amanda was considering was a high risk venture to fill her needs, and that it was fraught with difficulties.

'Have you considered the economic problems when you will have to spend time with your child instead of your job?' I asked. 'The father you intend to deceive will feel blackmailed and used and will be unlikely to form any relationship with his child. And he will have great bitterness towards *you*'.

I reminded her that her child would grow up without a father and would eventually have much resentment towards her for fulfilling her needs at their expense. From my experience as a mother, I knew that it is hard enough rearing a baby when there are two parents — being a sole parent must require heroic self-sacrifice, although I know it has been done and done well.

In a recent article, Dr Stephen Juan, a lecturer at Sydney University, quoted a child psychiatrist in America who theorises that there is a syndrome called 'father hunger'. Evidence suggests that the loss or absence of a father can 'result in children incurring severe, perhaps permanent psychological damage'.

I urged Amanda to think carefully about her decision. I felt she was suddenly overcome by panic and not facing the reality of what being a parent was all about. I asked if there was any way she could make a more positive effort to find the right man who thinks as she does. I also suggested that she expose herself to people with babies and small children, perhaps even baby-sitting for friends and relatives. Or she could do a little voluntary work in some situation where there were lots of young children.

Above all, I urged her to be as honest and decent as she could be with the man involved should she decide to go ahead. She should at least inform him of her intentions and give him a chance to agree or not to her proposition. That is the least she can do for her own self-respect, as well as his.

WE DON'T WANT CHILDREN

The choice not to have children is one which I see more often now than in the past. Couples who absolutely do not want children have an easier time than those whose decision is not so clear-cut. Being such an emotion issue, it stirs up many feelings and doubts which cannot be easily resolved. Ellen's letter was such a one:

'I am 33 and we have been happily married for seven years. Twelve months ago I became pregnant. This was totally unplanned as we had decided some years ago not to have any children. We were shocked and distressed and in the end decided to have the pregnancy terminated. I was not prepared, however, for the pain and guilt and loss I would feel and sometimes still feel, and now I am totally confused about whether I want a family or not, despite my earlier strong convictions about not having a family.

'My husband remains sure he does not and has spoken of a vasectomy to make sure we don't go through this trauma again. He understands how I feel and says he won't do anything until I'm sure of what I want and that if I do want children he won't say no. Most of the time I'm sure I don't want children, but other times the thought of being childless fills me with fear. Our real problem is that my parents have sensed my indecision and have been pressuring me incessantly to start a family "before it's too late". We told no one of my pregnancy or termination but they can't accept our decision not to have children and it's all they have talked about for months. This has only upset me and confused me more and my husband is furious with them. I need more time to decide what I want, but I don't know how to convince my parents to stop interfering and the tension between them and my husband is unbearable. Please help me.'

I told Ellen that she and her husband must do what they think is right for them at present, but not to take any irreversible steps just now while she is still so undecided. It is possible that they could change their minds in the future, but that would have to be their considered choice and no one has the right to influence them in whatever decision they make. The weight of evidence suggested that Ellen's husband did not want children. If he gave in to her wishes while still feeling as he does, he would surely turn on her every time there was any trouble or conflict. But before finalising their decision, I urged them to have counselling from a social worker at an obstetrics hospital. An objective viewpoint can often clarify our own feelings.

I urged Ellen to tell her parents to back off and leave her and her husband to make this very important decision without pressure from outside.

'But be kind as you tell them to keep out of such personal affairs', I said. 'After all, they may find it hard to understand that some people don't want to be parents.'

My last piece of advice was 'Keep communicating with your husband. In the present climate it is easy to create a rift between you, so keep up a united front.'

I WANT GRANDCHILDREN

The choice not to have children affects more people than the husband and wife concerned. Grandparents-to-be, or more appropriately, not-to-be, are often distressed and confused. Marge wrote to me because of this.

'I am a 66-year-old widow and for some time I have
been urging my only daughter and her husband to
start a family before it's too late. She is now 30. Last
week she finally informed me that they do not want
children, and I am totally devastated by the decision. I
would have loved a large family, but emergency surgery
after the birth of my daughter put an end to those
plans, and I pinned my hopes on grandchildren instead.
The thought of growing old without them leaves me
feeling very empty and lonely. I also worry that my
daughter will regret her decision when she is too old to

have babies. I would like to tell her how I feel, but am
very much afraid that she will resent my interference.
What do you think I should do?'

I told Marge that I understood how unhappy she must be over
her daughter's decision, but that she could not expect her
daughter to provide the family she had wanted and didn't have.
Unfortunately, we can't live our dreams through our children
and they can't live their lives in order to please us.

I also told her that her life would be empty and lonely only if
she allowed it to become so, or that she could use her warm,
nurturing instincts to reach out and enfold others who would
welcome what she had to give. With the changing pattern of
family life there are many young people who would love to have
a Grannie for their children, but who are deprived of this relationship for whatever reason. Love and caring need not be limited to blood-relatives only. The human family is a reality which
we are recognising more and more.

I suggested that perhaps she could offer her services to an
organisation in her state where she could be with children and
develop an intimate bond with a few of them. She would benefit
and so would they. I advised her against saying anything to her
daughter unless asked for an opinion and even then I urged her
to temper her answer to what was best for the younger woman.
Some people are not cut out to have children and it is wrong to
convince them otherwise. If Marge's daughter has regrets at
some later stage, she will have to come to terms with it and will
not be able to blame anyone else for coercing her to go against
her deepest feelings.

HOW DO I PROTECT MY CHILD?

This next letter from Patricia is timely and only one of a big
batch on the same topic. She wrote:

'I am rather confused as to how to deal with my
seven-year-old daughter's natural friendliness. She is a
beautiful child, outgoing and bubbly, and will talk to
anyone and everyone. I don't want to spoil this
trusting quality, or to worry or alarm her by

emphasising the dangers she can get into, but I'm so
scared her friendliness will get her into trouble. She
walks to and from school by herself.'

This is very much a problem of our times and I wanted to give
the most helpful answer possible.

'All caring mothers are as anxious as you are about this real
danger,' I wrote, 'yet no parent wants to dampen a friendly
child's spontaneity and make him or her suspicious or withdrawn. On the other hand, their safety has to be considered. I
think your seven-year-old should be accompanied to and from
school until she is a little older.

'But here comes the difficult part: for although you must tell
her about not getting into cars with strangers or accepting anything from them, you must also warn her against *anyone*, even
those she knows well and who may want to interfere with her
clothing or her body. For it is a most unfortunate and unpleasant
fact of life that most molesting of children happens in the child's
own home and from people who are close to them — uncles,
family friends, brothers and even fathers.

'It's a good idea to tell your little daughter that most grown-up
people are kind to children, but that there are a few who can be
very unkind indeed, and that no matter who they are, she must
not be afraid to tell them to leave her alone. You can do no more
than be reasonably cautious and watchful.'

RELATING TO YOUR PARENTS

Lillian was an older woman and her letter demonstrates the
long-lasting effect of a mother's unloving behaviour. She wrote:

'I am a middle-aged woman and ridiculous as it may
sound, my problem concerns the way I feel about my
mother. Everyone including my husband and my father
knows that she is a very difficult, critical, unloving,
narrow-minded person and a trouble-maker. Yet my
guilty feelings about not even liking her, let alone
loving her, are spoiling my otherwise happy life. Is it
too late for someone like me to ask for help so that I
can achieve peace of mind?'

It is never too late to look for answers or to try fresh approaches to old problems. It seemed that Lillian had good reasons for not liking her mother and if it were anyone but her mother who treated her as badly as she says, she'd have handled the whole relationship objectively. As it is, she is torn apart by conflicting emotions. A face-to-face discussion with a trained counsellor would enable Lillian to come to terms with the way she feels and the way she tells herself she ought to feel. It would help her to understand that it isn't compulsory to love your parents.

This letter is a good example of the far-reaching impact of a mother's attitude on a person's life. Despite Lillian's age, her unhappy feelings about her mother are affecting all her other relationships. She claims to be otherwise happy, but the mother-child relationship is so basic I have no doubt that some of the resentment and dislike is seeping into the way she relates to others. The guilt she admits to is enough to contaminate all her good feelings for anyone else.

The mother-child relationship is the closest you can have — it involves a genetic attachment which is deeper than any subconscious attachment of the mind. We all need to accept this as we are stuck with it. But we also need to accept it as a fact of life that some people are incompatible, no matter whether they are strangers or our mothers/children. It is then up to us to decide what is rational and make a choice.

Lillian needs to grant her mother the right to be who she is but in doing this she must free herself of any obligation to 'love her'. A few sessions of counselling will hopefully enable Lillian to accept her mother as she is, forgive her and then let her go. Even the fourth commandment only orders us to *honour* our mother and our father. It says nothing about liking or loving them.

Moira's letter was unusual but since it shows the far-reaching effects of the mother-child bond, it is appropriate in this section.

'My husband is 24 and was adopted as a baby.
Although he had a loving relationship with his
adoptive mother, he felt the need to know his natural
mother and finally found her. When he and his mother

first met they spent every day and night together. That
was fine at first, until it ran our lives. He forgot
everyone (even our baby) and we argued a lot because I
didn't agree with the way things had turned out. It
might sound selfish, but we are on the verge of
divorce. It's also tearing the other family apart.'

I replied, 'Your husband's behaviour is not unusual in cases
where mother and child are reunited for the first time since
infancy. There is an overwhelming need to be together to allow
the bonding process which should have happened at birth and
later to develop. They can't help the way they feel.

The desperate need to make up for lost years makes them
unaware of how deeply they are hurting those around them.
Usually this passes in a few months so perhaps you need to be
extra patient if you want to save your marriage.

It's clear that you need a bit of back-up and support at this time
so I urge you to get in touch with a Community Health Centre
near you or with Centacare, Lifeline or Family Life. All these
numbers are in the phone book. Talk to someone today.'

Margaret's mother is very demanding of her daughter's time:

'I'm married with two school-aged children. My mother
— a widow — lives near us in very comfortable
circumstances. She is physically quite active but
dislikes going out unless I accompany her, and as a
result, she sees no one except me. I go to her house
every day except Sundays and have little time for my
own family or any other interests. It's making me very
depressed, especially as we argue a lot, but she won't
hear of having visits from other people. When I've tried
to cut down my visits I've always felt guilty and can't
enjoy my freedom. My family think I give in to her, so
I get no help from them. What can I do?'

'You can begin to listen to your family's opinion and try to
realise just how pointless this situation is,' I replied. 'And it's as
damaging to her as it is to you. It's doing no good at all to your
mother to restrict her life to one place, one relationship and one

interest — herself. And it isn't even a happy relationship between her and you, is it? A lot of resentment is probably all that's left and it's blighting the rest of your life.

'So bring this dependence of hers out in the open. You're both adults and you don't have to pretend that everything is rosy. Give her the choice of widening her interests or of being lonely. If she refuses visits from anyone else, so be it. Be kind, but don't yield on the fact that your visits are going to be shorter and fewer. You can show just as much concern for her — and ease your mind at the same time — by ringing her up for a chat occasionally. Dismiss any guilty feelings. In the circumstances they are inappropriate. What you have done for your mother so far is over and above the call of duty. Your first duty now is to your immediate family and your mother comes second, and you must gently force her to see this for her good as well as yours.'

Sonia's letter was interesting in that it reminded me of the importance of touch for every human being and even more so for babies and elderly people.

'My mother has the idea that the more you worry over a person, the more you love them. I have told her I don't worry about anyone as it is a useless emotion and nothing is achieved. Now she has the silly idea I don't love her, which is rubbish, and is even thinking of leaving me out of her will just because in her estimation I don't worry enough. This hurts me because at a practical level I have always done everything to help her. I have been a good and loyal daughter, often helping far more than my siblings ever did. How can I convince her that it is the practical aspect which is more important?'

'I applaud your practical, commonsense approach to life, but must point out that this often needs to be balanced by a visibly loving attitude. Many people like your mother measure love by the amount of fuss being made over them. She can't help feeling this way — it is coming from an emotional deficit and not a rational part of her. So what she needs from you are more gestures of affection such as hugging and touching as you talk or walk by. Perhaps you are too matter-of-fact and she takes this as rejection. You are obviously better educated than she is, but you will have to meet her on the level she needs and understands. Even if you don't really love her, you will not be a hypocrite in showing love and compassion as a human being. Duty is wasted if it is devoid of love.'

BIRDS MUST FLY THE NEST

Mary wrote:

'My 18-year-old daughter has just told me that she's going to leave home because it's driving her crazy. She accused me and her father of being in a rut, of never doing anything "different", and says we've been too soft with her, smothering her with love and affection instead of being the firm parents she needed to give her direction and confidence. I'm so shocked and hurt by all this. We have always done what we thought was the very best for her and her two brothers. How can I win her back?'

I knew many mothers would identify with Mary.

'You haven't lost her. It's just that it's time for her to move out, and many children can only make this break by being aggressive about it. (One part of them really wants to stay!) If you had been short on affection she'd be blasting you for that. It's not rational and it's not personally directed at you, but only at the 'smothering ties' of childhood she now wants to get rid of. So let her go and help her struggle to be independent. It is only after she has become her own person that she can begin to see you and her father as real people and not just parents. Then you will find that you have not lost a daughter but gained a real friend.'

SINGLE MOTHERS

When I first began my column, a single mother was a rarity. Today I receive many letters from single mums, so many in fact, that I regard it as one of the major changes in society in recent times. This one is from Lisa:

'I am 24 and a single mother. Since my boyfriend left
me three years ago, I haven't been able to let myself
get close to any man. I feel I have been hurt once and
don't want to be hurt again. I loved and trusted my
boyfriend very much and thought he felt the same, but
when I fell pregnant he just changed. I always hoped
he'd love his daughter, but he never did. However, I
want to change for my own and my daughter's sake.
How can I forget everything that happened and get on
with my life?'

I had to tell Lisa that she can't erase the past — none of us can — but she can learn to leave this past where it belongs and live in the present. I know this is easier said than done, especially as she has a child to remind her, but it means the difference between a balanced life and one filled with resentment. Lisa's trust has been shattered and she has built a wall around herself as protection against further hurt. It's a natural reaction, but that wall will also keep away human warmth and contact and any possibility of finding genuine love. Unless we allow ourselves to be vulnerable as well as cautious, we can't experience life.

I felt that Lisa had become more aware of what she wanted from life and was ready to make changes, so a course to help her find what makes her tick would be a good idea. It would also put her in touch with other like-minded people who were searching for the same values she was seeking. I urged her to enquire at her Community Health Centre and find out what was available. She would also benefit greatly from joining a playgroup in her area where she would meet other young mothers and her daughter would enjoy the company of other children. By relating to women in similar circumstances, Lisa would get a feeling of support and companionship as well as a broader viewpoint. Our best lessons are learned from relating to other people.

This letter from Maggie shows a single mother with no sense of self. It demonstrates that the best thing a mother can do for her children is to be a person in her own right.

'I'm an unmarried mum with an eight-year-old
daughter. We live at home with my parents and we all

get along really well. The problem is my daughter. She 'hates' everything — her meals, toys, going to bed, everything. She cries and yells when asked to do something like picking up her clothes. She is always whingeing and says she is bored. She often has friends to play here, and goes to friends' places and generally you couldn't find a nicer little girl. She had a lot of illness last year and was in and out of hospital for six months. I blame myself because she is probably spoilt. She likes school and looks forward to going. She is bright and does well and I think she gets on well with everyone. She plays netball and goes to Brownies. When she gets angry with me she uses bad language and abuses me. I've tried smacking and punishing but she doesn't care. She gets on well with my family but seems to hate me. By the way, she has the same name as you — Kate.'

My impression was that this child had too many adults in her life and did not feel she had an exclusive mother-child relationship with Maggie. Her angry outbursts were an attempt to show her mother how she felt. The fact that she got on well with others both at school and at play reinforced this conclusion. It was clear that Maggie was depressed and that Kate was spoilt because her mother was uncertain in her role as a parent.

'She gets angry and frustrated,' I wrote back, 'because she needs you to be an effective mother and place limits on her behaviour. She also needs you to take responsibility for the fact that you are her mother above any other relationship.'

I felt that Maggie needed to have some sort of life of her own which is not easy since she is living with her own parents and probably reverted to being a child herself sometimes. And she was doing everything to make the child's life as full as possible while completely neglecting her own.

I reassured her that her daughter did not hate her. She was simply letting her know that she was unhappy with the way she was behaving as a mother.

'So do get out there and do something for yourself,' I said. 'Smacking is not a good method of child-rearing. All it means is that the mother has also lost control, and no child can relate well to that. Listening, really listening when the child wants to talk to you may give you a clearer picture of what is upsetting her so deeply.' I also urged Maggie to try Parent Effectiveness Training by enquiring at her nearest Community Health Centre.

Another facet of single motherhood is revealed in Moira's letter:

> 'Last year, my 17-year-old daughter became pregnant. I thought she was too young and immature to raise a child, but she insisted on keeping the baby, left school and found a job. Now her son is eight months old, she seems to have no feelings for him and refuses to look after his physical needs. She has left her job and spends her day moping around the house and talking to friends on the phone.
>
> I have taken leave from my job to care for my grandson, but much as I love him, I've had my years of childbearing and don't want this to be a permanent thing. What should I do?'

'Your daughter *is* too young and immature to raise a child,' I wrote back, 'but she was wilful in her choice and now she must be made to see her responsibilities. Push her into a corner by telling her the baby will have to be adopted out if she does not start behaving like a mother. (You don't have to mean it, but say it as though you meant it.) You will be teaching your daughter a valuable lesson if you make her see that she can't go on doing as she pleases and then letting others pick up the pieces.

Tell her you will give her support, but make it quite clear that she is the mother and that she had better begin to behave like one. This is definitely a case of having to be cruel to be kind.'

INDULGENCE IS NOT LOVE

Our relationship with our children affects every relationship they will ever have so its importance cannot be over-emphasised. Consider this letter from Louisa. I am certain she did not set out to harm her child.

> 'My five-year-old son started school this year and after a few weeks changed from a bright, happy child into a

sulky, withdrawn one. He says he hates school and it's
a battle each morning to get him to go. I'll admit we've
spoiled him. For ten years we thought we were going to
be childless and then he arrived. I know I can't have
any more so naturally he is precious to us. He has
always been precocious, a bit of a show-off and always
has to be the centre of attention, but I honestly
thought he'd grow out of it. He is teased and made fun
of at school and the other children refuse to play with
him, so that he comes home crying nearly every day.
We're very worried about him and wonder what is the
best way to handle this problem.'

I had to tell Louisa what I'm sure she didn't want to hear,
namely that the responsibility for her little boy's misery was
mostly hers. In the first place, indulgence is not loving. By
encouraging his precocious ways and pampering him, she had
turned him into a child who is disliked by other children.

'If you want him to become a likeable, decent human being
later on,' I said, 'you'll have to give him the tools he can use as
he grows up. You'll have to start a gradual unspoiling process,
otherwise he'll have an even harder time in later years.'

It's clear he has not been taught to give and take — he is too
used to receiving. I suggested that she start by explaining gently
that as people grow up they've got to learn some rules and stick
to them. I said it was OK to give in sometimes but not to give the
child everything he asks for. It was imperative that she only
reward him when he does the right thing.

'When he shows off', I said, 'keep the praise for his perform-
ance at a low key. But don't make the mistake of ignoring his
showing off altogether or he'll find other ways to gain attention.'

It would be a good idea to teach him to give sometimes and
not always take. Unless changes were made now he would
become emotionally dependent and would establish the 'spoilt
brat' pattern for life. And no one outside his home would give
him the loving 'strokes' for being such an obnoxious person.

'He needs to learn the consequences of his behaviour, to see
the cause and effect', I said, 'but whatever you do, try not to give

your son a sense of inferiority in your efforts to right the mistakes you have made. He still needs plenty of love and reassurance.'

I urged her to encourage him to invite some of his schoolmates home and to let him visit when asked.

The sad part of this letter is that Louisa and her husband believed that loving the boy was enough to make everything right. While it is true that love is of vital importance, too much permissiveness confuses a child so that they do not *feel* loved. Perhaps the feedback he is getting at school will be the best teaching experience of all. With his parents' support and goodwill and a more objective approach, it is not too late to reverse the child's negative conditioning, but if things don't improve, I suggested that they seek counselling.

Single mothers are not the only ones with problems in parenting. Children need the love and guidance of a father as well as their mother. As mentioned before, research has shown that there is such a thing as 'father hunger' where the father is absent or completely uninvolved or inadequate. Since, as we have seen, we learn to parent from the example of our own parents, it is usually those who lacked good role models in their own lives who fail in this relationship. Consider this letter from Gina:

'I can't get my husband to discipline our three children aged six, four and two. The eldest two are spoilt because their father gives them sweets instead of discipline. They swear and scream and never do as they are told. They run my husband's life. I can't seem to control them and feel as if I am heading for a nervous breakdown. My husband works during the week and goes surfing all the weekend which means I have the children nearly all the time. Six years of babies has already made me tired and cranky. Now even the youngest screams and hits me if he doesn't get what he wants. Their father does not believe in smacking them.'

While it was clear that the children had become a problem, I could see that this was only a symptom of what was happening within the family. One of the difficulties in parenting is that our own unresolved conflicts of a particular age are stirred up by our children when they reach that same age. Gina's husband had probably been brought up in a repressive environment which he could not accept, and now he was reliving that period through his own children by behaving, and letting them behave, in the way he would have liked to do when he was young. Now he was transferring the frustration and anger he felt against his mother onto Gina by refusing to back her up in disciplining the children. He did not seem to know what being father really means and their relationship was hardly a happy one with Gina in the role of the 'dragon' and with him as one of the children.

The problem was too complex for this family to solve alone and I urged them as a family to seek professional counselling as soon as possible. I was sure the children's behaviour would not improve at this point until Gina and her husband found an effective way of handling conflict, relationships and parenthood. I suggested that their doctor would refer them to a reliable family therapist, or they could ask at any large hospital.

WHY DON'T I LOVE MY BABY?

Although it may be difficult to understand how a mother could not love her baby, it happens often enough to warrant a mention. This letter from Rosie is typical of such letters:

'I can't talk about my problem to anyone else in case they jump to the wrong conclusion that I'm a neglectful mother which I'm not. But why can't I love my baby as much as I should? I never enjoy touching him or playing with him, and I only talk to him at mealtimes. I think he senses I don't love him because he cries a lot with me but is such a happy baby when my mother has him. Why am I unable to mother my own child? What can I do about it?'

'What you can do — and should do — is get help. No one is going to jump to any conclusions. It's quite obvious you are doing all the things that a caring mother does, but without the loving feelings, so find out what is blocking them.

'Perhaps you did not receive the mothering you needed as a baby. It's now recognised that some babies need much more than the normal range of touching and caring and even though they were loved dearly, are left with a deficit need. Or there may be unresolved conflicts in your life or with the child's father. Whatever the reason, a word with your own doctor, or someone who knows you and your son will set you on the right track for the help you need.'

I MIGHT HURT MY BABY

The urge some people feel to hurt their baby, sometimes severely, is more common than is realised. The reasons for these feelings are many and complex but it is good to know that help is just a phone call away. C.A.P.S. (Child Abuse Prevention Society) was originally formed with the aim of helping mothers in this predicament although it has now extended its services to include children who are victims of sexual abuse.

Here is Sally's letter:

'Please help me as I am desperate. I am a 24-year-old single mother of a 13-month-old son and I keep on having the feeling that I want to hurt him and even kill him. I don't know why I feel like this because I really love him most of the time, but when I get into these moods I am scared of what I might do. Sometimes I smack him really hard so that I hurt him and then I feel so guilty I cry for hours. I don't know why I do it. I must be a very wicked person to feel like this and hate myself so much I sometimes feel I should kill myself as well as him. Kate, please give me some hope.'

I hoped I could give Sally something to hang on to, when I wrote 'You are not a wicked person, and many more women than you imagine have these same feelings about their babies. The psychological reasons are too complex to be dealt with here, but they are related to your own early experiences and to the stresses in your life. You sound very depressed to me and that should be treated first of all, so see your doctor or enquire at one of the Women's Health Services in your state.

But the best help you can get is from contacting the Child Abuse Prevention Society (CAPS). Their 24-hour emergency number is (02) 344 7646. They are trained to deal with such matters and will give you all the understanding and support you want, as well as referring you to the nearest help group in your state. I urge you to ring as soon as possible. You can't go on suffering like this much longer.'

4

The Teenage Years

MOST PARENTS WISH their children could jump from the age of 12 to 21 without going through adolescence. If we are to believe even some of what we hear, this stage is like trying to find your way in a foreign country whose language you don't know, without a map, with no signposts and at night! Yet the many adolescents who move towards adulthood with little or no trauma, never make the news.

In the 50s in America and the 60s in Australia, young people were emerging as a separate group in our society, with their own label — teenager. The media had not recognised their growing status, but parents were already feeling the pressure, although at that stage it was mild. In my day there was no such thing as a teenager. You were a baby, a child, a girl or boy and then you were grown up and that was that. Family life gave the support and back-up it had always done, and letters from young people reflected a measure of stability despite the difficulties. Their problems were simple, their needs uncomplicated.

This all changed with the coming of the sexual revolution when teenagers took the lead in their search for total freedom. Children began experimenting with adult activities before they were ready to cope with the responsibilities these entailed. Too many regarded sex as little more than a baked dinner — eat it and forget it. This was rarely without its consequences and those carefree years between childhood and adulthood were lost forever. In those early years of my column, the 'generation gap' was a favourite expression and a much-used excuse for anything that went wrong between parents and children.

Looking back, I feel that too many parents relinquished their important role as parents and became even more confused than their children. This was a time when children lost respect for their parents — a loss which has never been fully regained. Without that loving support and strength to guide them through the rocky path of adolescence, teenagers either gave up on themselves or behaved in extreme ways as a means of testing their parents' love or gaining their attention. Young people need strong role models in order to define themselves.

The teenage years are a time of rapid change and much questioning of all that went before. There are changes in body shape, discovery of the opposite sex, strange new stirrings, the realisation that parents *don't* know everything — and pimples! Unresolved conflicts from childhood are stirred up and must be dealt with again, this time as a budding adult rather than as a child. The natural urge to spread their wings and leave the nest, vies with the desire to step back into childhood and let mum and dad do the worrying.

This is also the age when the need to belong to the group is so strong it leads to what is called 'peer-group pressure'. Young persons who feel good about themselves can withstand more of this pressure than those who feel insecure. Yet too many parents also succumb to this peer-pressure and opt out of their parental responsibilities. They are afraid to risk being unpopular by stating the truth as they see it. They don't remain firm in what they believe so how can they expect it in their children?

Our heady race towards total freedom has brought us to the end of the line. If we ask 'Freedom from what?' we find that it was a revolt against the harsh rules and repressions left over from the Victorian era, especially in matters of sex. I feel this had to come, and it was a healthy swing, but now the pendulum has swung too far the other way. Total freedom without responsibility amounts to abandonment, and the abandoned children of today are witness to this rejection. I receive far too many letters from people who avoid all responsibility and commitment and feel they have total freedom. The trouble is they can't understand why their lives are such a mess!

Real freedom comes when people feel they can handle their responsibilities and are not burdened by them. They can tell the truth and face the truth about what is important in their lives. In ancient societies they would have been the 'wise elders' who passed on the wisdom of their experience to those who came after them. Today, many of us have forfeited the right to guide the next generation. If we are confused, they will be confused and their children, and theirs again. It is an awesome responsibility but also a magnificent opportunity to meet the challenge!

Despite their apparent waywardness, or perhaps because of it, life is not easy for teenagers today. The changes in family patterns have undermined the security which was gained from that safe environment in the past. The bomb has taken over from witches and giants and monsters of our childhood stories as a fearful reality. There is an increase in violence and economic instability, and even going to the beach has become a health hazard! No wonder so many youngsters feel disoriented and hopeless. All the letters in this section portray some aspect of the problems faced by the younger generation.

IT'S NO FUN

Judy's letter was one of the most accurate descriptions I have read of the doubts and fears so many teenagers go through.

'I am 13 years old and my problem is that I really hate myself. I am always fighting with someone. I've just lost my best friend because I was bitchy. One part of me kept telling me to stop it, but I just couldn't help myself. I also had a row with my mother who says I choose weird clothes. I get jealous of everyone and everything and my moods chop and change like the weather. I'm not pretty and I'm not ugly either. When I go with a guy I always seem to want to go with someone else. There's only one guy I really like, but then I'm not even sure I do. I'm in trouble at school because I'm behind with my homework. I'm in such a muddle I don't know whether I'm coming or going. I've even thought of suicide. My emotions drive me up the wall, God help me. My parents don't know I feel this way.'

In my reply I said it wasn't the end of the world, although it might feel like it.

'When you're thirteen,' I said, 'your moods swing up and down like a yo-yo. One week everything goes wrong, the next week your friends love you, you get the highest marks for assignments, and go shopping for clothes with your mother who confesses to some weird fashion mistakes of her own when young.'

I added that at present everything was happening too quickly. Her body was changing — hormones which are making her a grown-up woman and forcing her to leave her carefree childhood behind, are zapping around and causing all these confused feelings. She feels grown up one day and the next day she wishes she was a little girl again. She does not know how to deal with all these conflicting emotions.

I suggested that she should apologise to her friend for her behaviour. It is never too early to rectify mistakes we make, and if we don't learn to do it we can destroy all of our relationships.

The impression I had of Judy was that she didn't belong anywhere, there was no direction in her life. She was like a ship without a rudder. Even her rebellious feelings had no foundation. It was as though she had nothing to go for and nothing to rebel against. I urged her to talk to her mother and if she really felt she couldn't, suggested a favourite aunt, a teacher, a good friend or even a friend's mother who might listen and understand. I said it helps to talk things out when you are looking for answers, as it often clarifies how you are really feeling and what is the core of your problem. I also suggested that pouring out your thoughts and feelings in a diary was helpful and so was talking to yourself and being your own best friend.

Self-talk is very powerful in either a positive or negative sense, depending on how we use it. The positive words we say to ourselves are wonderful therapy. Negative words can destroy our self-worth more than anything else. We have the choice whether to be for or against ourselves. I advised her to accept her changing feelings, the bad moods as well as the good ones, to acknowledge them all but not to make a habit of gloom and negativity. A cheerful attitude can become as much a habit as a discontented one.

Judy had ended her letter with 'God help me' which led me to suggest that turning to a Higher Power would surely give her strength and guidance.

WHY AM I BORED?

I receive many letters from young people who are bored and for whom life has no meaning at all. They are a sad reflection on our times. So much is available to youngsters today in the way of entertainment and leisure that they are overwhelmed by choices. It has become 'not cool' to be excited about anything. Mandy's letter is an example of this malaise:

> 'I'm a 15-year-old girl and so fed up with life I could die. I am in year 10 at school but lately I'm falling behind in my work because I can't make myself study. I have a few good friends and we all go out at weekends. I'm not allowed to go out week nights, but they are. The problem is that even when we are out I get bored and wish I was somewhere else, but I don't know where. I'd like my life to make a difference but I don't see how. Nothing makes me feel good anymore. Is there anything I can do to feel less bored? If this is all there is to life, it's not worth living.'

Boredom is an unhappy state and can have many causes. The main one in Mandy's case is lack of involvement in anything outside herself. Most people hate being bored and try to avoid it at any cost, some through artificial means which include drugs, alcohol, over-eating and frenetic activity. They discover soon enough that this is not the answer. Others find their own way of overcoming it through work, meaningful relationships and interests and causes they believe in. Sometimes they become addicted to dangerous sports as a relief from boredom.

In our world of technical achievements, everything is geared to give us input — television, radio, movies, magazines and newspapers. We are used to having everything poured into us with no effort on our part and as soon as it stops we are at a loss. This is only natural because if what we take in is not balanced with what we give out, our lives get out of kilter and become static. What we need to do is break that cycle of boredom with action of some sort.

My advice to Mandy was: 'Use your imagination and think of what you'd do if anything was possible. Then choose something and *do it*. Your schoolwork can become an exciting challenge instead of a chore. Do something you may not have thought of in the past. Join a musical society or learn to play an instrument. Take up bushwalking with a group, or Tai Chi. Joining up with a group which does something constructive for the community as well as socialising can be fun and very fulfilling. Anything which involves you. Remember that involvement creates interest and enthusiasm will come in the doing.

'Another 'cycle breaker' is to think of all the things you love to do and the things which leave you with a sense of wellbeing after you've done them. Write them down. This will stimulate your creativity which is a good antidote to boredom. Spending a few hours with a friend at a funfair or going down the slippery dip in the park can bring back some of the delights you felt as a child and give your spontaneous feelings a boost.

'Or you can tidy up your room and clean out a few drawers. You can sort out your clothes and fix up those that need repairs such as buttons and hems. You can decide to give away those that you no longer can use. You can bake a cake or ring up someone you haven't seen for a long time and arrange a meeting. Or you can go for a long walk and notice, *really notice*, things along the way which you normally take for granted — the playful puppy that rushes out to greet you, the flowering peach trees across the road, the old lady who smiles at you as she goes past. That is the way we get our energy flowing outward so that fresh energy can flow in and create a balance.'

Human beings were not made to be static. We are dynamic and need to express ourselves or the life force becomes stagnant. And that is what boredom is. When we sit in a chair complaining that we're bored, we are surrendering to everything that is negative. We are relinquishing all control over our lives. In effect, we are saying: 'I'm helpless, unable to make anything happen.' This is not true. Being alive is a marvellous opportunity to make things happen and so prove you exist.

Boredom in youth can become a search to find a solution. If you don't do anything about it but let it continue, it will eventually become a habit and by the time you are 35 or so it will become uncontrollable depression. Then you will be looking for excesses to give you relief, which of course, they won't.

I also advised Mandy, and offer this advice to anyone else who wants to get out of a rut, to try to learn something new every day. It can be a new word or something you read whether it be at school or in a book or newspaper or magazine. If you do this *every* day, you will feel you are in touch with the world again.

Life is full of opportunities. There are so many experiences that can be unexpectedly meaningful. 'So get moving and let the Force be with you, and life will be worth living again.'

WHEN FAMILIES ARE NOT SUPPORTIVE

Sometimes a problem assumes such proportions that a person is overwhelmed and thinks of suicide. Because of their youth, teenagers are more vulnerable than older people who have life experiences and past successes to back them up. Tragically, many of the teenagers who write to me can't envisage any solution except killing themselves. This letter from Sharon was one of the saddest letters I have received. And yet her spirit shone through so brightly, I felt there was cause for hope.

'My mother kicked me out when I was thirteen. She said she didn't want me and didn't need me in her life so I went to live with my father. After a year I was a different person. I had low self-esteem and felt depressed so I went back to live with my mother. After a couple of weeks I felt so hopeless I tried to kill myself with two packets of Dispirin because I truly felt I would be happier dead. Funnily enough I was saved by a lady I didn't even know. After coming back from hospital she and her husband took me to live with them and treated me like family. I've never felt so loved and secure in my life. Her children treated me like an older sister and she and I were like a real mother and daughter.

'Two years later we had an argument (only the second in all that time) but it hurt me so much I ran away to live with my mother, who I thought had changed. She begged me to come home so I moved back (I still don't know why I did it). Now I have a good job but I miss that family so much I could just die. My mother is treating me like garbage again. When she gets drunk (which is most of the time), she starts arguments that eventually lead to her telling me that I'm a nothing and that she wishes I would go back and live with my father. I can feel myself going off the tracks again. I am so confused. I wish I could see that family again but the mother isn't talking to me. I really need someone to talk to but I don't like burdening my friends. Please don't suggest counselling. I went for a year after I tried killing myself and they thought we were delinquents and treated us as such. I just wish I could see my other mother — the one who has been the only real mother to me. I love her so much.'

The pain in this letter touched me deeply. Here was a child who had been so bruised emotionally that she would consider killing herself. I could understand why. There was no one she could trust or turn to. From past encounters with mothers such as Sharon's, I deduced that her mother was self-centred and immature and resented having to care for a helpless baby and now a 'demanding' teenager. She (the mother) was a dependent personality and because she had never been mothered she had no idea of how to mother her own daughter. She turned to drink to blot out her own pain.

Sharon's father was a kindly man but weak, unreliable and two-faced. She always hoped he would become the true father she wanted, one with whom she could feel safe and protected, but his weakness and indifference disillusioned her hope. I did not need intuition to tell me that these parents individually and together were most destructive for Sharon and would ultimately lead to a tragic end for this girl. The only glimmer of hope I saw was her spirit, her lack of self-pity which might have been excused in the circumstances, and her capacity for giving and receiving love. People who have never been loved usually find this impossible to do.

Her perceptions and awareness were acute but emotionally she was still a child and in need of support and guidance. It was two weeks after she returned to her mother's house that she wrote her letter to me. I wished she had given an address so that I could have replied at once. Her letter and her reply would take the required four to six weeks before they appeared in the magazine and I was concerned for her. I knew she was at a crucial stage of her development when she needed a good role model if she was not to turn out like her mother — or try suicide again. My intuition told me she had been badly damaged in her early years and was beginning to feel she didn't deserve to be happy. This led her to behave in a way which messed up her life. I wondered if she had subconsciously jeopardised her happy life with the 'family' because of her distorted belief in her unworthiness. Unless this belief system was reversed now, I knew there would be no hope for Sharon.

The one solution I could give her was this: 'To write a long, honest letter to the only real mother you have known, that kind lady who saved your life. It doesn't matter what the argument was about — tell her how sorry you are and ask to be forgiven and taken back into her family. You must also forgive any hurt that was done to you. That family was the only place where you have found solace and love and you would be crazy to give it up. If they are the loving, compassionate people you say they are, and which I don't doubt, they will not allow one quarrel to destroy the relationship they had with you. On no account must you stay with your mother, nor would I advise you to go with your father. You were unlucky to have found indifferent counsellors. Fortunately they are not all the same.

I prayed that Sharon would choose to change the old, destructive patterns with which she had been programmed and fulfil her potential for happiness. I also hoped that the 'other mother' would pick up the magazine and read the letter. She could not fail to recognise the details and perhaps make some move towards the girl she had come to love as a daughter.

I sometimes think of Sharon and wonder how life has turned out for her. I can only hope that her story ended happily.

GOING OUT WITH BOYS

'Going out with boys' is the predominating problem I read in my mail from teenage girls and their mothers. Trisha's was such a one. Her letter was written in red ink in a rounded childish hand with the i's dotted with tiny circles instead of a dot.

> 'My parents seem to think that at 14 I am too young
> to go out with boys. Lots of boys have asked me out
> but I have always put them off.'

The reason she was writing to me was that now there was a boy she'd really like to go out with and she was tempted to do so without telling her parents who would surely stop her. She asked: 'Do you think I am too young?'

How easy it would be, I thought, if I could give an arbitrary age at which a young girl suddenly became old enough to 'go out with boys'. The reality is that going out with a boy isn't a matter of how old you are but how ready you are for this step. A girl is ready if she has mixed a fair bit with both sexes at home and in other homes, at school, clubs and in social activities. Then both the girl and her parents can feel confident that she is able to take good care of herself.

So Trisha's idea of having secret dates with boys her parents have never met only points to the fact that she is *not* ready. I advised her to take this boy home, to see him for a while with the rest of the crowd and then see how her parents felt about her going out alone with him. It was probably not the answer she wanted to hear but it was the only one possible in the circumstances. Most parents might not approve of a steady boyfriend at the tender age of 13 or 14, but I'm sure they would not object to a girl going to a movie occasionally with a friend who happened to be a boy or with a group of boys and girls.

THE OTHER SIDE OF THE STORY

The next letter is from Robert and was unusually interesting in that it gave another point of view. I usually hear from girls who complain 'He was after only one thing.' He began:

'You often have letters from girls asking how to say
"no" to a boy without chasing him away for good, but
you've never had a letter from a boy asking the same
question about girls. Believe me, it's harder, really,
because a boy can more readily look a fool when he
says it. I'm 18, still at school (I do my final exams this
year), am popular and am told I'm good-looking. At
present I am going out with a 16-year-old girl whom I
like very much. We have a lot in common and I enjoy
tennis and surfing with her. But lately I can tell she'd
like to go further than I know I should for both our
sakes. I'm no prude, that's for sure, but how can I get
out of such a situation without looking stupid, and
making her feel even worse? This has happened a
couple of times in the past year with other girls. I've
discussed this with a few of my friends and they agree
with me — sometimes they have sex because the girl
wants it, yet they'd rather not.'

Robert sounded like a intelligent, sensitive young man.

'All you have to do,' I said, 'is to be honest with this girl and
any other girl, as you have been in your letter to me. At the right
moment, say "For both our sakes we're not going any further".

'I assure you you won't look a fool — in fact, there are many
girls who would admire and applaud you and who would give
anything to meet a real man like you.'

THE COLD, HARD FACTS

When the letter which follows reached me, I was surprised. I
don't often get this kind of feedback. Kristine wrote:

'Recently I read of a 14-year-old girl who went out with
boys behind her parents' backs and got pregnant. As I
have been through it all I thought I might help other
girls if I told them about it. Firstly, telling your
parents may seem impossible — I thought mine would
kill me — but they were terrific. I was fifteen and ten
months when my son was born, and then I had to go
through the trauma of seeing my boyfriend charged

with carnal knowledge and in gaol for a night and a
good behaviour bond for two years. And it was hard
looking after a baby. I wanted to prove I was a good
mother and thought I knew all about it, but looking
after your own is not the same as looking after
someone else's for a short while.

'You're with the baby all the time, changing nappies,
feeding him in the middle of the night, trying to cope
with his crying and his tummy-aches as well as looking
after the flat, wash and cook. My friends were still at
school so I didn't have anyone my own age to talk to
about my problems. They would talk about their latest
boy or the dances they were going to and I used to get
jealous and wish I could have a bit of fun like them.
You miss out on the best years of your life and it's
hard on the baby too as it knows when its mother
doesn't know what she is doing.

'My boyfriend and I married when I was 16 but we
were divorced later. My son is six now and I'm coping
better but although I love him very much, if I could be
14 again and know what I know now, none of this
would have happened. So be careful girls. It's no picnic.'

I could sense the maturity gained through hardship and pain,
the lessons learned and I hoped that now life was kind to
Kristine.

INFATUATIONS — DO'S AND DON'T'S

This next letter touches on an important aspect of teenage infatuation. I receive many such letters from worried mothers.

'My 16-year-old daughter is mad about a boy of 18 who
wants to visit all the time. We've cut down his visits to
two a week, but resent having him at all. We feel she
is too young but don't want to put our foot down in
case she starts to meet him secretly. Although he is a
nice boy, he's not what we'd like our daughter to
marry, but she is talking about marrying him at 18. We
tell her to concentrate on her studies for now and then

have lots of friends both male and female and see a bit
of the world before she marries. She says it's her
business not ours. What can we do?'

This mother's anxiety is making her jump to conclusions which might never occur. I tried to reassure her by pointing to the 'facts' as opposed to her assumptions.

'Your daughter talks of marriage now,' I said, 'in an attempt to be grown-up, but this does not mean she will feel the same about him when she is 18. The worst thing you can do is make this boy unwelcome and treat him unfairly or with resentment. This will make her jump to his defence, and then it will be the two of them against you. A forbidden relationship is always more desirable and exciting.

'But if you treat her as a friend and allow her to talk freely without preaching or judgment, she is more likely to let the infatuation run its course without having to hang on simply to defy you. And while he is there in your home with her, at least you will know what is going on. Your love and support and honest communication are the most effective tools you have.

I WANT MORE FREEDOM

One of the most common problems teenagers write about relates to freedom — freedom to go out when they want and with members of the opposite sex. This next letter from Ellie was sent to me by her mother with a short, accompanying note. 'I found this in my daughter's room while cleaning and 'I give you permission to print it. Incidentally, my daughter goes out as much as she likes in the daytime. She also goes dancing three nights a week.'

I put the letter to one side as I felt uneasy publishing it without Ellie's knowledge. Two days later Ellie sent me her own letter. The letter her mother had found was a first draught.

It is not often I have the chance to read two sides of any problem and it was enlightening to see both points of view.

'I am nearly 14 and lately have been having a few
problems with my parents, the main one being that I
don't go out that much. I have lots of friends who go

out together. I want to go roller-skating with them at
night (my boyfriend goes too), but my parents won't let
me go. I do pretty well at school and I'm not a bad
sort of kid, but I'm desperate as I hate sitting at home
doing nothing while my friends are all having fun. How
can I convince my parents to let me go out more?'

I felt that Ellie was enjoying a fair amount of freedom but it was clear that she perceived her friends as having more and she hankered after the same privilege. She sounded responsible enough, but her parents' concern was understandable. I said it wasn't easy being 14 just as it wasn't easy being the parents of a 14-year-old. I felt that the only way to prevent resentment and misunderstanding from building up on both sides was by honest discussion as to what they all consider a fair set of rules and an agreement on trust. They must all be able to trust one another.

I urged Ellie to tell her parents how left out and lonely she feels sometimes — and they may confess just how much they worry about her safety and welfare. If she tells them how confused she feels lately, they'll probably admit that they are feeling confused too about doing what is best for her. If they can establish a 'climate' where it is safe to be honest, they could not only solve this present problem but would set a pattern of behaviour which will serve them well in the future. I asked her to consider how much her parents must love her and be concerned for her safety to be risking being so unpopular with her.

The next letter shows a mother genuinely trying to understand and her willingness to work things out in a loving way.

'My 15-year-old daughter thinks I'm old-fashioned and
unfair because I won't allow her to go out alone in the
evenings with her girlfriends the same age. I trust her
as I know her to be mature and sensible but I feel
anxious about it unless she's going with people I know,
will be accompanied home, and can give me a definite
time to expect her. I have to say "no" to just going out
to a disco or a milk-bar "on spec". She says I'm ruining
her life, but has agreed to listen to your point of view.
Would you let a daughter of this age go out alone at
night more or less to see what turned up?'

Personally I wouldn't and I told her so. It's not that all young people she may come across when she's out are not to be trusted, but that a 15-year-old girl does not yet have the ability to judge whom to trust and whom not to trust, nor the ability to handle tricky people and situations.

'Your daughter will be developing these abilities now if she has the opportunity to mix with both sexes in the ordinary life of work and play,' I answered.

This mother sounds caring and aware and I was sure her anxiety would be lessened and her daughter's boundaries allowed to expand if she left the way clear for her to become involved in school and local club and church activities, and by encouraging her to bring friends home. I advised her to focus on understanding her daughter as an individual and not as a problem teenager which she was not.

FATHERS AND SONS

I can't explain why I get more letters from girls than from boys. I can only put it down to the fact that boys don't talk about what is bugging them as much as girls do. Geoff did not write to me — his mother did.

'Until about a year ago my husband and eldest son (we have three) got on marvellously. Now they seem to do nothing but row, and all I do is try to keep the peace. Sometimes it looks as if each hates the other and that troubles me greatly as we have always been a close and loving family. My son is a good boy and often talks to me saying he just can't help flaring up at his father, and my husband is a good man and a good father. Perhaps now that his final exams are over, Geoff will settle down a bit. I hope so. I can't take this warfare any longer.'

This is a familiar situation. Most fathers and sons are in conflict at some time or other. It's all to do with subconscious competition and a boy's need to assert his independence. Sometimes mothers contribute by being overprotective towards sons, creating jealousy in their husbands. I suggested to this mother that she could help by backing off and not taking sides.

'In many ways it is a healthy sign that your son can spar with his father in this way,' I said. 'It means he feels safe in his father's love. All children need to vent their feelings of frustration in a socially acceptable way. And the best place for this to happen is in the home where they are basically assured of their parents' love and can feel safe without fear of being rejected for their outspokenness. Frustration which is constantly repressed often breaks out in violence and other anti-social acts.'

Of course, I am referring to the occasional outburst and not a constant aggression. Whenever this happens, professional help is indicated but it did not seem necessary in Geoff's case. A strong and loving father is the best role model a boy can have.

CLOTHING RULES

While it is true that teenage rebellion provokes many of the conflicts I hear about, there are times when the rigidity and lack of awareness on the part of parents reminds me that no problem is ever one-sided. Consider this letter from Debbie:

'I'm 12 and quite happy except for one thing. My parents insist that I wear clothes which they think are right but which make me feel like a freak. My school uniforms are down over my knees while all the other girls wear them short. In winter my mother insists on knitting me cardigans which make me look like an old lady. I'm teased and laughed at, but all my parents say is that they know what is best for a 12-year-old. They don't. Can you please help me?'

I also receive many letters from young girls who feel the need to shave their legs or underarms, or to wear a bra but are forbidden by their parents. If only they would realise how devastating it is for children to feel freakishly different from their friends. To my mind it is one of the most painful experiences a child can go through and is a form of abuse. In most cases it is the parents' fear that the child is fast growing up which makes them try to deny it by forbidding any signs of approaching adulthood. I always urge these girls to show them their letter to me, published with my reply, in the hope that an outside opinion will change their parents' attitude.

The other side of the clothing debate is illustrated by Emma's letter — dressing in a provocative way:

'I am 16, still at school and have a problem which is really upsetting me. My father gets angry because I love mod clothes and mini skirts. He says I try to look too sexy. I can't stand to dress in pretty-pretty clothes or look like a goody-goody two shoes. I am an excellent student and otherwise get on well with my parents who are very understanding. I have lots of good friends, both boys and girls. But I can't make my dad see that there is nothing wrong with wearing modern gear and looking sexy. He's always saying that it's not right to dress in a way, that it turns boys on even if I don't do anything about it. How do I convince my father that it's not what you wear but who you are inside that's really important?'

I could see Anna's point of view as well as her father's and I wanted to let her know I understood the confusion. At the same time her letter brought out clearly what I wrote about in the introduction to this chapter — that responsibility is intrinsic to freedom. I felt Emma was not aware of her own subconscious urge to 'turn boys on' as though it was a game in which she could win. I felt her father's fears were more than justified, and that she was selling herself short. Here is my reply:

'What is it you really want in a relationship and in a boyfriend? Ideally, what sort of boy do you want in your romantic life? You sound intelligent and perceptive and at 16, your natural youth and beauty are sexy enough without being blatant about it. You have other attributes which are attractive — your warmth, enthusiasm and humour which come through in what you say. Boys look for these qualities as well as sex so don't underestimate either the boys or your own worth.

'In any age there is a line beyond which fashion becomes more than just dressing attractively, and becomes a flaunting of your sexuality. If this is what you do, the boys you will attract will only want you for your body. By dressing in a provocative way you can't blame them for thinking your body is all you have to offer. Surely you want a boy who will accept you as the total person you are?

'Since your parents are understanding, why not have a heart-to-heart talk and come to an agreement which is fair and pleasing to all of you. Keep in mind that it's more desirable to look sexy while still retaining a little mystery and promise.'

TEENAGE DRINKING

Penny's letter left me feeling sad. I often wonder how things have turned out for her.

> 'I am 16 and very shy. For the past six months when I go out with blokes I have a couple of drinks so I won't feel so shy. Sometimes I get drunk and they take advantage of me. I only began drinking because all my friends did at parties and I thought it was cool. And now I can't stop. Every time I go to discos I get drunk and at home I sneak glasses of wine out of my father's bar. My friends say I drink too much. I want to stop but I can't. Could you tell me another way to overcome my shyness without drinking?'

I wondered why so many girls regard shyness almost as a crime. I wrote back that there is nothing wrong with being shy when you're young, in fact, it's very appealing and attractive. Far better to grow in self-confidence as you get older than to be brash and overconfident too soon.

At sixteen it was only natural that Penny should be interested in boys but not to the exclusion of all else and not in the way she was doing. This was the age when she should be enthusiastic about learning new things, developing her mind and skills and therefore her whole personality. Sex was a part of this learning but only a part. The only way to overcome her shyness was to develop her full potential as a human being and to respect herself. Her present behaviour was destroying all her self-esteem and sabotaging any attempt to feel good about herself.

I suggested that going out in groups with boys and girls was the best way to learn to interact socially in an easy way. And I also said that it was not 'cool' to go around in a state of stupor and allow boys to use her. The best thing she could do would be to ring Alcoholics Anonymous and enlist their help and support in kicking her habit. 'That's all it is just now,' I said, 'but if you don't put an end to it, your life will be ruined.'

DRUGS

Sophie's letter is one of many I receive expressing the same problem:

'I am 16 and my boyfriend is 23. My parents used to let him come to our place and take me out as long as he got me home on time and no drink driving. Then they found out he was on drugs and also had another girlfriend, so they stopped me seeing him. I started sneaking out at night to see him but they found out and told me not to see him for a few months while we worked ourselves out. I love him and he says he loves me so we ran away to another state. Now my parents don't want anything to do with me. He can't get a job and my parents wrote and stopped me claiming the homeless children's benefit. They'll have me back, but only on their conditions. I want to stay here.'

I found this letter very difficult to answer. I did not want to 'lecture' yet Sophie needed my honest opinion.

'It seems to me your parents are not unreasonable in their expectations of how you should behave and gave you options which you knocked back. You are making decisions with your feelings which you ought to be making with your brain and are mistaking the strength of these feelings for wisdom.

'What your parents have and you do not yet have is experience of life. You are caught up in the romance, excitement and attraction this boy has for you. Believe me, the boy you find irresistible at 16 is very different from what you find attractive in a man at 18 or 20. I advise you to take things more slowly while you achieve the maturity which will help you choose a partner with whom you can have a happy future. At 23, your boyfriend is selfish, immature and irresponsible to persuade someone of your age to leave her home when he has absolutely nothing to offer. Face the facts — he is unemployed, unfaithful and on drugs. Your parents' assumption that someone on drugs has impaired judgment and little chance of leading a normal life unless he is strong-minded enough to kick the habit, is correct. Unless he can do this, your life with him would be a downhill slide as his will be.

'My advice is that you, and this boy, if he wishes, should go back to your parents' home and have a round table talk with them. You need to express what you feel, but you also need to listen to what they have to tell you. You must all make some agreements which you must honour. Remember it was you who broke the original agreements which were set up by your parents to protect you. They love and care about what happens to you. You still need their guidance and protection. You will not get that from your boyfriend.'

AM I GAY?

The one topic on which I receive the same number of letters from both sexes is the subject of sexual identity. Fears about sexual inclinations disturb and confuse a lot of young people. Here is Sandra's letter:

'I'm desperately worried that I may be a lesbian. I'm 18 and attend a teachers' training college. I have normal relationships with boys but I'm attracted to a very kind, affectionate woman of 35 who is married and has two children. There's nothing sexual in it. All I want her to do is love me and cuddle me. I often daydream that I'm part of her family. I've felt like this about different women since I was about nine. My parents were divorced when I was seven and I lived with my mother who remarried and had two other children. What's wrong with me?

It was as clear as daylight that Sandra wished this woman was her mother and that she had longed for mothering from women in the past. There's nothing wrong or odd about that. Many people, particular those who lacked good mothering as children feel a great need to be mothered as adults and into old age.

Women often find it indirectly in their friendships with other women, in a good continuing relationship with their mothers, or from tender husbands and lovers.

It was my guess that Sandra had probably missed out on the mothering she would have wanted when her mother's attention and affection was turned to her children in the second marriage. This had left a gap in Sandra's life which had never been filled.

'You can't expect the cuddling you want from your friend now that you are no longer a child,' I said, 'but the kindness and affection she is giving you are the grown-up substitutes for it. This relationship can give you what you want most at the moment, the feeling of being loved and thought well of — if you will simply make up your mind to relax and let it.'

Although Sandra's problem may appear similar to this following one from Nell, the motivation is completely different. While Sandra's is caused by a deficit need, Nell is going through a developmental stage where loving someone of her own sex and hero-worshipping is a stepping stone from childhood to hetero-sexual love. Here is her letter:

'I'm a 15-year-old schoolgirl and I think I'm in love with my French teacher. You'll probably think I'm silly, but I often dream about her and during the holidays I feel lonely because she isn't there. Just before the Christmas holidays when I found out she wasn't coming back to our school this year, I broke down and cried a lot. I just wish I could be like her and be always with her. I'm really scared I'm a lesbian.'

I could reassure Nell that just because she loves another woman it doesn't mean she is a lesbian. I felt that probably what had really scared her was the intensity of her feelings. It's a fact that in the middle of their teenage years youngsters often ident-ify strongly with someone of their own sex who is quite apart from family and friends. If a person is lonely or there's a difficult family situation, that relationship becomes very important to him/her. Hero-worshipping is a safe way of coming to terms with our developing sexual feelings. Of course, I don't think Nell is silly but I was sure her tears had more than one reason.

When you're young and vulnerable, as all teenagers are in vary-ing degrees, emotions are always close to the surface.

'This love you feel,' I wrote back, 'is a kind of bridge towards heterosexual love, that is the love you'll feel for the opposite sex.' I hope she was reassured.

This letter from Craig is only one of many letters on this subject:

'I am an 18-year-old male and scared that I am a homosexual. For about four years I have had sexual feelings towards different men but have never had a girlfriend nor have I been interested in girls. I haven't told anyone how I feel and there is no way I could tell my parents as it would break their hearts. I do not have anyone else to talk to and am quite desperate to be rid of this problem.'

I discussed Craig's letter with an expert in this field, a Profes-sor at one of our larger hospitals. He felt that nothing in this letter added up conclusively to this young man being homosex-ual. I learned that most boys between the ages of 14 and 18 are confused and searching for their identity especially their sexual identity. For most of them, on the way to becoming heterosexual they hero-worship members of their own sex and look up to them as models of how they'd like to be themselves.

I felt that Craig's lack of interest in girls may have stemmed more from lack of opportunity, than from his natural inclination. My impression of this young man was that he was shy and socially inexperienced. In other words, he hadn't given himself the chance to find out about who he really was.

I went on to say that if he did find that he is homosexual, there is no need to feel so desperate — accepting himself, whatever his leanings, is the one important thing he could do. However, his aversion to homosexuality would give him a very strong motivation to change, so his best bet would be to see a doctor or community health counsellor who could refer him to specialist therapy if it was needed.

5

Loving and Being Loved

NO WORD IN the English language is more open to misunderstanding and abuse than the word 'love'. Love has many expressions — there is love of parents for their children, love of God, brotherly love, romantic love, and of course, love of self. Unless we love ourselves we cannot love anyone else yet most of us are unaware of this truth.

When we speak of love we mostly refer to romantic love and it is this kind which seems to create the greatest conflict. No doubt this is because 'love' is used to describe a condition or state of feeling which is often anything but love. Passion, ardour, infatuation, lust, excitement and obsessive need are often interpreted as love, and while they may be a part of being in love they are not loving in its truest sense.

Every human being needs to love and be loved, and as I read between the lines of the letters I receive, I sense that lack of self-love is the cause of many seemingly unrelated problems. When people talk about love, what they have in mind is romantic excitement, living happily ever after, and the end to all their problems. Having found the 'right person', life will now settle down to perfect contentment, all their needs and aspirations satisfied. This is the accepted fantasy, the romantic ideal that most people have been yearning for since Adam and Eve.

This myth has been perpetuated and enhanced more especially in recent times by songs, poems, stories, television and films. Currently, the idea of love has been used and exploited by advertisers who persuade people that their dream can become a reality with the help of their beauty aids, drinks, cigarettes, garments and so on. The result is that many are brainwashed into believing this is possible and they feel like failures if it doesn't happen that way.

There is no doubt that romantic love is exhilarating and joyous, but its very intensity precludes it from lasting at that level for long. Real love is an ongoing process between two people who are willing to grow together and contribute to each other so that their relationship deepens. But no matter how much two people love each other, they are individuals and perfect communication and harmony often do not exist. I feel that we have come to expect too much of romantic love which invariably leads to disappointment. Like so many things in modern life, romantic love has become another 'instant commodity'. If it doesn't give immediate joy and gratification, throw it away and try again with someone else.

I often hear from girls and women who are so caught up in the love myth, they will fall for and even marry the first man who says 'I love you', only to discover too late that they have nothing in common. Just as sad are the letters from men who feel used and exploited by their wives.

Love is one of the most confusing of human feelings. In fact, it creates some of our worst problems. Because of the impossible expectations where love is concerned, many of the letters I receive are about the stress and pain of love gone wrong.

IS IT LOVE?

One of the most often asked questions is: 'How do I know if it's really love?' This letter is from Sandra:

'I am 23-years-old and would like to know how you can
tell when you're really in love. I've known a guy since
I was 15 and had a school crush on him. We hadn't
seen each other for seven years, yet I've never forgotten
him. I went on a date with him recently and slept
with him on this occasion and once previously. I can't
seem to get him off my mind. He says the loveliest
things to me when we're together and wants to

continue seeing me. How do I know how he really feels
without pestering him or presuming we have a so-called
relationship?'

I replied that the only way to find out how he really feels is to
take it quietly and continue a relationship which lasts over a
period and concentrates on more than just sex. It is impossible
to know anybody well over a short time. Even though she may
find him unbearably attractive, it takes more than that to know
what a person is really like. I reminded her that by sleeping with
him so soon, she had already created a commitment on her part.

There are no sure-fire tests which tell us when love is real or
only a crush, but really caring about someone like we do about
ourselves is a true sign of real love. Sandra and her boyfriend
had the beginnings of a relationship. Now she must be patient
and see if it would develop any further.

Debra wrote:

'I've been going out with a boy for eight months. I love
him very much but I just don't know whether to
believe him when he says he loves me. He's very good
to me and respects me, and is always saying he loves
me. But does he or will he change?'

Debra was asking for the answer to an eternal question which
has no guaranteed answer.

'You're asking whether this love is the genuine article that will
last forever. But there's no certainty about people's feelings for
each other — and never can be. You can only enjoy for your own
sake the feelings he has for you now, which are clearly loving
ones. All he asks in return is that you love him, too. So what do
you have to lose by believing him? Let go of this "heavy" attitude
(it's caused by insecurity and anxiety), and enjoy!'

LOVE vs FRIENDSHIP

I receive many letters from girls who are good friends with a boy
but who feel they are falling in love with him and want something more. In most cases the boy seems satisfied with friendship without commitment. It is stating the obvious to say that

love can grow from friendship and when it does, it is the most enduring and rewarding love of all. Of course, there is no guarantee that this will always happen, but it is possible if the relationship between the couple is allowed to develop at its own pace without forcing it. Sometimes people do not recognise this slow-blossoming love because it was not 'at first sight'.

Debbie wrote:

'I am 19 and have known and liked a guy for two years. We are good friends and we both like spending time together and with other friends. We can talk openly to each other about anything and I value that, but I am falling in love with him and want more than friendship. The only trouble is that he thinks we are just good friends.'

I sensed that Debbie and her boy had all the makings for a good, strong love. They had compatibility, common interests, openness and the ability to talk on an intimate level. The fact that they could enjoy a wider circle of friends as well as their own company, also told me the relationship was not obsessive but stable and balanced. Despite all these things going for it there was no certainty that he would fall in love with her as she had done with him.

'Very often when a girl falls in love as you have done, the relationship changes', I replied. 'From being a good friend, she becomes possessive and manipulative. She tends to "crowd" him which sets off his alarm bells and all that was good between them turns sour. So give him emotional space, and he is more likely to like you more and more. There are subtle ways of letting him know you like him in a special way.'

I also suggested that she lead a fulfilling life apart from him. I urged her not to give up her friends, to follow her interests and be happy in what she does. By being interested and interesting you seem to draw other people to you. But it must be genuine and not a means to an end. If the romance blossoms, well and good. If it doesn't, the girl has expanded her vision and her skills and relationships so that she has gained a lot from her experience.

LOVE BLOSSOMS SLOWLY

There is more to Beth's story than appears at first reading — and it is interesting as well!

'Men have resented the fact that I have a mind of my own, and because of this, several romances have ended badly. Only one man seems to understand me. He has been in love with me for years and we have slept together many times. He keeps asking me to marry him but I've always refused because I'm not in love with him, but he won't take 'no' for an answer. Whenever I break up with another guy, he's still there. Do you think I should marry him anyway? I like and respect him and miss him when I'm not with him. He says he has enough love for both of us.'

'Maybe he has enough love for both of you, but it would be unfair to marry a man you don't love. However, if you take a closer look at your feelings for this man they may be deeper than you think. Sometimes love begins suddenly, but it can also grow so slowly that you hardly recognise it when it blooms. Now it's about time you gave this possibility some thought, and it could be that your romances end badly not because you have a mind of your own, but because you are too opinionated. My guess, though, is that you care more about this faithful guy than you'll admit even to yourself, and so you subconsciously sabotage the possibility of romance with anyone else.'

FEAR OF LONELINESS

Joanne wrote:

'I have never had a boyfriend and now at 23, I am going steady for the first time. He says he loves me and talks about us getting married, but it worries me that we are poles apart in every way. He is not very well-educated and can't carry on a conversation about anything that interests me. The only thing he's interested in is sport which I can't stand. But he is

the only man who has ever said he loves me and I'm
scared that I'll reach middle age and won't find a man
who will feel that way about me.'

Joanne's fear is very common. Many people fear that love will
die, or that they'll never be loved again. 'You can't build a marriage on the sole basis of avoiding this fear,' I wrote.

It was clear from her letter that she did not love him nor did
she respect him or rejoice in his company. Her words were a
put-down from start to finish and no love between two people
can survive that kind of contempt. I suggested that since what
we are all looking for in the long run is to be loved, this boy
deserved to find with someone else what she felt she was unable
to give him. I could only hope that this, her first experience of
being loved, would build up Joanne's self-image to the point
where she could be patient, rather than obsessive, about finding
a partner with whom she had more in common.

LOVE SHOULD NOT BE SELFISH

Rachel's letter is an example of how actions that are anything but
loving, are interpreted as love.

'A boy I went out with last year is now going with
another girl. He often comes to see me and says he
misses me. He says he'd be very upset if I went out
with anyone else. But he won't take me out at all
because of his other girl. I wish I knew how he feels
about me. I think he still loves me, or why would he
be jealous if he didn't?'

It is true that we often see what we want to see and Rachel is
seeing love where none is there and never was.

'Love has nothing to do with it,' I said. 'He's just a dog in the
manger. He doesn't want you himself but he'd like to stop
anyone else having you. As this means keeping you in an
unhappy, lonely state, it's obvious he doesn't give a damn for you
as a person. Do go out and build other friendships and tell him
to push off. If he gets upset, it's too bad.'

This letter from Nick shows how family jealousy can harm relationships. He wrote:

> 'I'm a 21-year-old bachelor who has always found it
> hard to make friends with girls. However, a few months
> ago I finally got my act together and asked a girl in
> my office to go out with me. She accepted and
> everything was great until last week, when, at my
> mother's insistence, I took my girlfriend home. It was a
> disaster. Not only did my mother take an instant dislike
> to her, but also she seemed unable to keep this dislike
> to herself. She criticised everything about my girlfriend
> — and in a very underhand way — and now my girl
> is so upset she refuses to go out with me again. I'm so
> wretched, I feel like moving out and never talking to
> my mother again. But my father died five years ago
> and she doesn't have anyone but me to look out for
> her.'

'Your caring attitude towards your mother is commendable,' I wrote, 'but the kind of spite she showed can be so shattering and hurtful that I think your first action should be to comfort your girlfriend. If you were getting on well before this, she is probably only keeping away from you for fear that you're taking your mother's side. You must make it absolutely clear you're not and that you don't share or approve of your mother's attitude. And I don't think your mother's rudeness should just be excused and passed over. If you intend to live at home for a while yet, it's really crucial to your happiness that your mother is at least courteous to your friends. I feel you should put this to her as a condition of taking anyone home — and of continuing to live there. Your mother doesn't sound too happy in herself — she may be jealous of your happiness, or scared this girl will take you away and she'll lose you. A few more friends of her own might help to solve that problem.'

Robin wrote:

> 'Since I started going with my boyfriend, I have lost
> every other friend I had. He is very jealous and

possessive and won't let me see anyone else, even other girls. I only go out with him at weekends and a couple of nights a week because he often works late, but he always rings me up. I think he does it more to check up on me than to talk to me. The other night I went shopping with Mum and was out when he rang and he was awful and wouldn't speak to me all day. The girls at work say I'm crazy to put up with him but I don't want to lose him. Can you think of a way to make him more reasonable?'

My answer was frank.

'It isn't going to be easy to get an unreasonable fellow like this to see sense. You can try but I'm inclined to agree with the girls at work. You are crazy to put up with this man's behaviour. You have to take a very tough line with him, for one of these days there's a fair chance you'll have a great big bust-up and you'll wake up to find that your life is very empty indeed.

'However deeply two people love each other, they cannot remain forever so completely wrapped up in each other that there is no room for friends and acquaintances. Your boyfriend has to learn to trust you and to share you with your friends. If he's that jealous now, he'd be ten times worse if you settled down with him permanently. You wouldn't have a moment's peace of mind. And neither would he. Tell him firmly that on the nights you don't meet you are going to visit friends or see a movie or whatever. If he doesn't like it, too bad.'

SHYNESS CAN BE MISINTERPRETED

I don't receive as many letters from men with problems of love as I do from women but David's was such a one.

'I'm a bachelor aged 20 and very shy. My father died 12 years ago and I still live with my mother. I have never had a girlfriend but there is a girl in my office who I have taken out a few times. I am desperately in love with her but am unable to show how I feel or make any advances to her. Even putting my arm around her is impossible for me. I am sure she must be getting sick of me and I don't want to lose her.'

I could see that easy affection and touching might be difficult for him as so far he wasn't used to that kind of body language with people. But that didn't mean he could not learn.

There he was with all that emotion churning around inside him, leaving her to guess what she meant to him. Moreover, he keeps wondering about how she feels and could be making a big mistake by imagining that she is getting sick of him.

'For a start,' I replied, 'why act as if you and this girl can't even talk? She could not possibly have overlooked the fact that you're shy,' I continued, 'and yet she has accepted invitations to go out with you more than once. So take courage and start talking about how you feel — gently at first.'

Once he could bring himself to talk about his feelings it would be a lot easier to act on them.

My last words of advice were: 'Switch off that critical tape playing in your head and go with your intuition.'

LOVE IS BLIND

Moira wrote:

'My 18-year-old daughter has fallen for a man who's nearly 40. He has had a broken marriage, two broken engagements and several failed business ventures. He is charming, but is clearly unstable and not, as my daughter believes, just the victim of bad luck.

'My daughter is a girl who needs lots of love, but I doubt he has any to give her. How can I make her see this? She is my only daughter and I am distraught.'

'Your fears are understandable,' I wrote back, 'and his track-record is not too bright, but your daughter could easily be one of those women who love someone they can "rescue", and for whom being loved is precisely this feeling of being needed. So what may seem a one-way relationship to you, could be completely fulfilling to her. It may turn out that she needs more from a permanent partner than this man can give her, but it takes time to find out how strong relationships are. If you oppose it or try to make her end it, you run far more risk of her rushing to his defence and wanting to "save" him than if you let her find out for herself whether or not he meets her needs.'

SEARCHING FOR IDEAL LOVE

Sometimes it is not the lack of love which is the problem, but the quality of love. When I read Tess's letter I realised she was searching for a deeper meaning to the act of love, something more than the meeting of two bodies, however rapturous that union may be. It seems to affect women more than men.

Tess had been married to Robert for four years and had a daughter of three and a son of ten months. She said she loved her husband but couldn't get through to him on a deeper level. He just wouldn't let her get that close. Tess felt secure, he was a good man and she didn't want to hurt him. But she felt she needed a deeper relationship. This was not enough for a lifetime. She asked me 'Should I break away now so that I am free to meet someone I can really love?'

It seemed to me that Tess was looking for an ideal kind of love which is very rare. It isn't an instant magic thing, either. In fact, it can take almost a lifetime to build. So if a deeper relationship was possible for her, it was within the marriage waiting to be developed over the years ahead. Even if Robert appeared to be aloof, this really wasn't saying his love was shallow, only that he couldn't show it. She could try to help him here by showing her love for him — women seem to find it easier than men — and this would help him respond. She could also talk to him about her deepest needs, and ask for what she wants. Perhaps she is expecting him to guess and he never will.

She needs to recognise that she has the concern, respect and affection for him that are the solid foundation of deep love. So instead of asking 'Is this all?', she could add up the advantages she had and build on them. I suggested that perhaps she was waiting for him to make the first move in sharing his feelings. By being more outgoing herself she could pave the way for him to follow her example. This would be putting into practice the old counselling dictum: 'Give your partner what you would like to receive', or, in other words, 'Do unto others as you would have them do unto you'.

ADULTEROUS LOVE

Our need to be loved is so great, it is sometimes all too easy to be misled by words which are, in reality, the very opposite of love. Consider Jan's letter:

'I am a 16-year-old girl and am seeing a 28-year-old married man who has a three-year-old son. He continually talks of leaving his wife to marry me. I am still at school and I am intimidated by his wishes.

My parents don't know I'm going out with him and they would be furious if they found out. I know he loves me and that I can trust him because he tells me he loves me and I know I love him, but I don't want the responsibility of his child. What should I do? Should I tell my parents?'

I did not like disillusioning her, however ...

'Just because someone tells you he loves you, does not mean he does or that you can trust him. In years to come "I love you" from a man who really loves you will be words to cherish, but at present all I can say is that words are cheap.

'A person's actions are the measure of his love. If he really loved you, he would not be trying to deceive an innocent, inexperienced girl who is still at school. He is not considering you at all but thinking only of himself. If he can't show loyalty and caring for his wife and child to whom he has a commitment, how can you expect him to care about *you*?

'The fact that you feel intimidated by his ideas and that you can't tell your parents is a good indication that this relationship is all wrong and can bring you nothing but unhappiness. Yours would not be the first story I have read where this has happened.

'Tell this man to go back to his wife and child — and tell your parents about him. Then, with that weight off your mind, enjoy your girlhood. These lovely years pass quickly enough.'

Love is the most healing force in the world, of that I am sure. But when we behave selfishly and without responsibility, all in the name of love, the results can be tragic. Here is Janet's letter:

'I started sleeping with my husband's mate and it turned into love, even though that's not what we wanted to happen. I also have a baby to this man. Only he and I know the baby belongs to him. The problem is I have this desperate desire to be with him all the time. I need him so badly I cry myself to sleep at night. I know he loves me and wants to be with me because he tells me constantly. Should we move in with each other and put up with the flak and hurt all the rest of the people involved? (I have three other children.) Or do we give up and forget this ever happened? I have feelings for my husband, but this is not love like I feel for my lover.'

'It was irresponsible of you both to start an affair in the first place,' I replied. 'Your strong feelings don't necessarily prove you're in love — it sounds more like a bout of sexual attraction and little else. The secrecy and excitement of an illicit affair is lending added intensity to your feelings. When you and your lover are living together on a day-to-day basis, the intensity will cool, as it must, and you'd be left with what? A shattered life for your husband and children, and resentment and guilt for yourself. I have counselled many women in a similar situation to yours and have heard their regret and anguish at the wrong choice they made.

'You played his destructive game. This man has nothing to lose, as you do. (You don't mention if he has a wife and children.) Are you prepared to give up your husband and children? Is this man worth such a sacrifice? I don't think so.

'You need to sit down quietly and make a reasoned choice rather than an emotive one. Imagine what it would be like now and in five years' time if you stayed with your husband and what it would be like if you left. Don't just think of all the good or all the bad in each case. Does your lover want to marry you or are you only desirable while off limits? The fact that you have "feelings" for your husband is a giveaway. The very real loving you have for him is overshadowed by the passion of your infatuation.'

I felt that my sharper-than-usual answer was justified. In the first place she had asked for my advice and I felt obliged to give an honest opinion. And despite her 'crush' I sensed her mixed feelings. Secondly, I am receiving so many letters on this same theme and have read so many stories of lives being destroyed by a passing urge that I must tell the truth as I see it.

As I said at the beginning of this chapter, 'love' is the most abused and misused word in the English language. Every sexual stirring is *not* necessarily love.

THE FIRST LOVE IS SPECIAL

Cathie wrote:

> 'I was desperately in love with my first boyfriend and don't think I ever really got over him. I'm 22 now and soon to be married. I love my fiancé very much but am filled with doubts as to whether I'm doing the right thing in marrying him when I still think of this other boy. Should I contact my first boy in case he's the one I love best?'

'First love goes very deep and is always remembered in a special way,' I wrote back. 'And doubts and backward glances just before marriage are perfectly normal too. Try to keep in mind that your first boy was in another time, another place — and should be left there. There's every chance he's changed too — engaged, married, or in love with someone else now. Any memories of past love, whether sad or happy, are a positive factor. They've helped to make you the loving person you are now. Learn to live with them, but don't try to relive them. Try this little technique which may 'complete' that part of your life. Look at a photo of your past boyfriend (or picture him in your mind), and tell him how much he meant to you and how you remember him with deep affection. Then say goodbye to him in any way you feel like doing. If doesn't matter if you cry, tears can be healing, but make the parting final and clean. Then you will feel free to give all your love to your fiance and the other will be just a happy memory. Try it anyway — it usually works.'

SINGLE PARENTS REMARRYING

The next letter from Pamela illustrates very clearly what happens when love is measured out and compared.

'I have a three-year-old son whom I love dearly. His
father disappeared when he heard I was pregnant and
now I'm glad he did as I know I didn't really love him.
I'm to be married soon and we have agreed that my
son will live with us. But I'm getting worried that my
husband-to-be really resents the child. I notice a hurt
expression on his face when I show my love for my
son. I love my fiancé very much, but I love my son
more. Could this lead to trouble when we marry?'

'Yes it could,' I answered, 'if you continue to measure and
compare your love in this way.' I felt there was no competition
between her love for her child and the man, unless she created
it. There is room in everyone's heart to love their spouse and
children — and many other people as well — not more or less
than each other, but differently. In my reply I said that if there is
really a hurt reaction from her fiance at times, this could be
because she showed her love for the boy, but neglected to do so
for the man. And he needed it just as much, but he had to accept
that her child was part of her and her history.

Love where there is no compassion is anything but love, yet
many people are deceived. They see what they want to see and
ignore the signs. Julie's letter was one of these:

'Ever since I divorced my husband six years ago, I have
been very lonely. Recently I met a man who says he
loves me and has asked me to marry him. I love him
too, but the problem is he wants me to leave my little
daughter with my parents as he says he doesn't want
to share me with anyone, not even her. I adore my
little girl and it would break my heart to part with her
and have her live with someone else even though I
know my parents love her very much. But I'm scared
to give this man up. I may never find another man
who would love me as he does.'

'I'm sorry to break the bad news,' I wrote back, 'but I don't
think this man loves you at all. Love without compassion is not
love, and anyone who demands that a parent give up a child, is

lacking both compassion and simple decency, as well as sensitivity. And without these qualities, what love can there be?'

I told her I could not make her decision for her, but asked her not to allow loneliness to ruin any chance of her future relationship with her child. I said I felt she was selling herself short by thinking this was her last chance to meet a man who would love her. It was all a matter of having a little more patience and the belief that a kind, loving man would come into her life.

MY LOVER IS MY BOSS

'My girlfriend works in the same firm as me, and has a more senior position. In fact, she is in charge of part of my work. We have no problems about this but our colleagues in the firm are always making snide remarks, implying that I'm working for promotion by going out with her. I am 32 and like my job and love my girlfriend who is 29. How can I stop these remarks and innuendos?'

'There's no need to', I replied. 'It's only teasing. If it were meant maliciously they'd say it behind both your backs, not to your face. Still, this change in the relative status of men and women at work is happening everywhere, and it does sometimes challenge a man's confidence and self-esteem — that's why you're a bit sensitive about the remarks. However, since you say it presents no real problem in your relationship, which is what really matters, you can both afford to treat all the remarks with humour instead of anxiety. You could even use the best deflector of all — agree with them cheerfully.'

TELLING YOUR CHILDREN YOU'RE IN LOVE

'I'm 45, divorced, and have two teenage daughters. I have now fallen desperately in love with a younger man. There is no question of marriage and we are very discreet — I would never allow him to sleep overnight at our house. But somehow I feel ashamed of letting my daughters know about this rather adolescent phase

I am in at present. Since it's so hard to keep it from
them because I'm so happy inside, do you think it
would matter if they knew?'

'Personally, I don't,' I said. 'I think it would be good for them
to know that you're an ordinary human being, who needs to love
and be loved and who can lose her heart in a romantic way,
without losing her head and ignoring responsibilities.

'They may, of course, be critical rather than understanding
simply because, at their ages, they'd tend to see falling in love as
inappropriate for anyone over 25. You know it isn't, and it will be
a useful experience for them to learn.'

PRISONER OF LOVE

Paula's letter demonstrates an aspect of love which I see all too
often in my counselling. She wrote:

'I think my husband loves me too much. He can't do
enough for me, helps with the baby, brings me presents
and sends me flowers. When he comes home from work
he likes to hold me close or have sex. He changes
completely if I want to go out on my own and gets
very upset. It's nice to be loved so much but his love
seems very selfish. It's as if he's frightened I'll leave
him for someone else if I go out. Please help me.'

'You've put your finger on the reason for your husband's terrific
concern for you — his great fear of losing you', I replied. 'It
would help you both to get this fear out in the open and overcome it. Otherwise it will grow worse and before you know it,
you'll begin to resent being treated as a prisoner, even a
cosseted one. Perhaps you'll find that someone important to him
in the past left him and he is terrified that history will repeat
itself. But he needs to find out that jailing you is far more likely
to drive you away than to build up his trust in you and your love
for him. You will need patience and compassion to reassure him
of this. Professional counselling would help you both.

LOVE IS NOT CRUEL

Consider this letter from Betsy. She was 15 and was 'desperately in love' with Chris, a 20-year-old man she was living with.

'He has a terrible temper, but always convinces me it's because of something I say or do. He often hits me, but is very sorry afterwards and tries to make it up to me by being Mr Wonderful for a little while. Then something else sets him off. He never tells me what it is so I can watch myself and not do it. Sometimes I feel I'd like to leave him because he hurts me so badly, but I love him so much and I know he loves me. I have no one to talk to about this. Please help me.'

I wondered why at the tender age of 15 Betsy did not have any family to turn to. It was clear she was looking for affection and would even put up with this ill-treatment to get it. It was equally clear that there had been physical violence in her family and she assumed that this was what love was all about and what she deserved. It was sad that the physical abuse she was enduring and the emotional damage she was being subjected to, was all in the name of love! The saddest part was that if she left this man she would most probably repeat this same pattern in every relationship because she would go on being attracted to and attracting men who ill-treated her. The only way to change the pattern would be for Betsy to have counselling which would help her see what was causing her to accept such abuse and turn her life around.

It seemed incredible that she could think she loved someone who beat her so cruelly and that he loved her, but in her deprived state it was understandable. Being 'close' to someone who beat her sometimes was better in her eyes than having no one at all. Until she changed her idea of what a decent relationship was all about, she would have no objectivity to choose someone who would give her a different life. To do this she would have to learn to love herself first of all.

SHOW SOME COMPASSION

Another effect from an abused childhood is illustrated in the next letter from Tom:

'I'm involved with a 22-year-old lady for whom I care very much. My problem is that she refuses to enter into a long-term relationship with me because she fears intimacy and commitment. She has revealed to me that she was sexually abused when she was 17. We also have problems communicating with each other what we really want and feel. I think counselling would be of little use as it was previously unsuccessful. What can we do to work through these problems?'

'It sounds as if your girlfriend, because of her disturbed background, has built up strong defences against relationships for fear of being hurt,' I answered. 'These defences usually start early in a family situation, and the episode of sexual abuse reinforced her fear of getting close to anyone. You need to tell her that unless she can talk and unbend and share her life and her thoughts and feelings, there is no relationship at all. If she is only prepared to have superficial encounters, she will never get any of the wonderful rewards that a close relationship brings. Since fear is the basis for her behaviour, talk gently to her. Let her know that although she has been hurt before, not everyone is the same, and that you won't let her down.

'If her hurt is too deep to trust you, ask her to ring the Child Abuse Prevention Service (CAPS — 24-hour telephone service is (02) 344 7646) and talk to a specially trained counsellor who will help her come to terms with her past trauma. Another option is that you and your girlfriend use each other as counsellors by talking about your deepest feelings and thoughts. This will deepen your understanding, as well as bringing you closer.'

6

Having an Affair

UNTIL THE END of the seventies, most of my mail relating to affairs was from distraught wives whose husbands had strayed. Those marriages usually ended in divorce. Nowadays, our changing values and opportunities have made it easier for women to have affairs, and an affair does not necessarily mean the end of a marriage. In fact, it can sometimes save a failing relationship by forcing a couple to face their problems.

Despite our greater tolerance in sexual matters, an affair is always a profoundly painful and traumatic experience for both parties and often for the 'other man or woman', as well. Naturally, the children involved in such triangles always suffer.

The reasons for having an affair are many and varied and often inexplicable but in my mail I have found that one cause predominates: the couple has not developed a common language which they both understand. It is better known as a lack of communication. By communication I do not mean idle chatter, but a couple's ability to be open and frank about their feelings, common interests, anxieties and worries, as well as their hopes, their joys and their hostilities. They can be angry with each other openly, and they can laugh together. This sharing of mutual feelings creates an intimacy which is even deeper than sexual union, however ecstatic that may be, but this intimacy cannot develop without clear communication.

Without words, pride, wrong assumptions and apathy take over until the rift is too wide to bridge. The inability to express feelings and to understand what the other is saying, leads to boredom, another real cause of affairs. If the relationship is in a rut, the partners look for other ways of breaking the monotony outside the married state. What starts off as a mild flirtation adding a little spice to daily routine, ends up a full-blown affair.

'A rough patch' in the marriage is one of the most common causes leading to an affair that I read about. Instead of taking the time and effort to look at what is wrong between them and talking about solutions, some people initiate an affair and for a while they can forget about their problems as they are swept up in the excitement and 'romance' of the new. There is no doubt that the feeling of being infatuated or 'in love' as they usually describe it, is a peak experience which is a boost to the system. What they don't know is that it cannot last in the routine of day-to-day living. Some people become so addicted to this 'high' that they move from partner to partner. But until they have resolved the difficulties which sabotaged their marriage, they will take the same problems into any future relationship.

If only they could put all that energy into their marriage where it would do the most good, they could revive and strengthen it beyond their expectations.

ADDICTIVE AFFAIRS

Lynne's description of her affair confirmed my view that sex can be an addiction as hard to shake off as any other dependency.

'Twelve months ago I started an affair with my boss. Both of us are married and there was, and is, no question of either of us leaving our legal partners. We decided we'd stop the affair when we came back from an interstate trip (I'm his secretary), but it's gone on and frankly, we both enjoy it. He doesn't seem to mind deceiving his wife, but I hate deceiving my husband. I am worried and nervous all the time. If my husband knew, it would be the end of my marriage. My boss says it's worth the risk of being found out, but I'm not so sure. I really don't know why I am writing to you but there's no one I can talk to about it. It's like a drug. You get hooked on it and would like to break the habit if you had the guts.'

My reply was what I felt she needed to hear.

'You really know what you should do — if you don't act now, your life will certainly be ruined. If you had any idea of the pain and trauma a break-up would bring on your loved ones and yourself, you'd get out of this situation fast. You write as though you have no say over what happens to you, but you do. We all have the gift of free will and it's up to us how we use it. Every addict, whether it be of drugs or sex, reaches a point where they must choose to stop or be destroyed. You have reached that point.

'Your boss is a selfish and egotistical man who is thinking only of himself and his own pleasure. He has no thought of what he is doing to you. He is using you as a sex object, nothing else. Break off the affair and get another job. You can tell your husband this job has become unbearable as the boss is too demanding. Consider as well that you are not simply addicted to your infatuation with this man, but also to the old habit of saying 'yes' when you want to say 'no'. You are used to being dominated.

'Now find the courage to do what you know you should do. Your whole future is on the line, so act — you don't have a moment to lose.'

AN AFFAIR OF THE HEART

This next letter from Tess shows us that sex is not the only component of an affair. An affair can be on the emotional level alone, but because the feelings involved are more fundamental, it can be even more painful when it ends. She wrote:

'Six months ago I had a kind of an affair with a
married man for four months. He was the first man I
had ever looked at since I married 19 years ago. We
didn't have sex although we both wanted to, and when
it got too hard to resist, we stopped meeting. It has
left such a sad gap in my life, and makes me feel so
guilty. I love my husband, but not in the same way
that I love this other man. Will I ever get over it?'

Although not an affair in its strictest sense, giving up a relationship which gave emotional fulfilment can leave a sense of loss as deep as any fully-fledged affair. Yet it can be turned around and used to make a marriage more satisfying. The affair has pinpointed the gaps which can now be filled.

I felt that Tess would get over this crisis more easily if she could stop looking at this friendship as a minus — as if it took away some good things she already had.

'Can you not look at it as a plus?' I asked. 'It confirmed that you are lovable and attractive, which you must have been doubting to have been drawn to the association in the first place, and the outcome shows you are both loyal, stable people who put your commitments first.'

FORGIVE AND FORGET

Pam wrote: 'My husband is a quiet family man, or at least he was until he went on a brief business trip overseas, and had an intense affair with a woman in her forties — he's 37. He came back full of guilt, jumpy and bad-tempered and told me the truth. I accepted his unfaithfulness because there's no question of his seeing her again and he assures me he felt no emotion for her — he was simply overwhelmed by physical feelings. We've made love since and he was his usual, gentle, considerate self. But in every other way he's totally unlike himself — restless, discontented, snappy with me and the children, finding fault with everything at work and at home. He has mentioned that "things will have to change" several times. It's breaking my heart and the whole family is so unhappy.'

What I could see was that in this intense encounter, Pam's husband discovered a freer, more aggressive and adventurous aspect of sexual behaviour than he's so far shared with Pam. It's left him feeling guilty and confused about what to do with his newly-revealed sensuality. Just now, he seems to be using this new energy rather destructively — lashing out at the steady, gentle routine he's been used to at home and at work. Where he can and should use it constructively is, of course, in bed with his wife. I urged her to do all she could to encourage an imaginative, more active approach to sex. He needs to see this as a healthy part of his nature, even if he regrets how he made the discovery. He can't repress these feelings any longer and shouldn't have to. But if he can't share them with Pam, he's likely to share them in unloving encounters with other women or vent his frustration in anger at work and at home.

'You already appreciate his gentleness,' I wrote back, 'Now learn to appreciate his other side — his dashing boldness.'

Wendy's letter shows how necessary it is to forgive — for her own sake as well as his.

> 'I have been married for 18 years and have three small
> children. My husband and I communicate well, or so I
> thought. I have just found out that he has been having
> an affair with a young girl 16 years his junior for two
> years. He told me he was in love with her. We have
> since moved to another state to start again. As far as
> he is concerned it is all over and should be left in the
> past, but I find I can't forgive and forget. Everything is
> good between us except this, as I can't seem to handle
> it. I have been to a counsellor but she says to put it
> all behind me. I find that hard to do. But I want to
> save my marriage.'

'Of course it's hard to forget,' I wrote back. 'Your trust has been destroyed, your confidence shaken. It is only human to feel betrayed. But your husband has shown most sincerely that you are more important than the affair, to the extent of moving to another state with you. Unless you can regain your faith and forgive him completely, you will ruin your marriage, your health and all you have gained. The counsellor you saw did not go into your feelings deeply enough. All that hurt is locked up inside you eroding your peace of mind.'

I was sure Wendy had never given vent to her rage and hurt and she needed to do that before she could let go of them for good. But that would have to be done in a safe situation. She could punch a cushion until she felt a sense of release, or polish the car or do an exercise class, all very physical acts which release blocked energy. I suggested a counselling service in her area. I could reassure her that once she had let go and really communicated with her husband about her feelings, as frankly and honestly as she could, her marriage would be stronger and better than before.

WHEN WIVES HAVE AFFAIRS

Most of the letters I receive regarding affairs are from women whose husbands are straying. Occasionally the tables are turned and a bewildered husband writes to me. Ted was repentant as well as hurt.

> 'I found out my wife was having an affair a few
> months ago. I realise I have taken her for granted and
> given her a hard time for years and I blame myself in
> some ways. She stopped seeing this other man and says
> she still has a lot of feeling left for me. But she seems
> half-dazed and doesn't show me the affection I'd like.
> She seems to be comparing me to this other man and I
> don't seem to match up to him. I'm so upset I can
> hardly eat or sleep. I love her and don't want to lose
> her but do you think if I threatened to divorce her
> she'd turn to me more? And should I tell our children
> about the affair? They have no idea what happened and
> seem to be blaming me. She is deeply ashamed for her
> lapse.'

I reminded Ted that by his own admission he treated her badly for years and actually drove her to seek love elsewhere. I told him how cruel and stupid it would be to think of threatening her with divorce and exposing her unhappiness to her children. If he wanted to salvage his marriage, he would have to treat her with gentleness and real concern. He really had to believe what he said about his own selfishness and unkindness and act accordingly — just saying it wasn't enough. And he would need patience. After all, she gave up a man she loved to save her marriage and may not feel loving towards him for some time.

'The more love and compassion you show her, the greater the chance of renewing your relationship,' was my parting reply.

Simon's wife had also walked out. He was younger than Ted and more desperate.

'Help me Kate, as I am desperate. I am a 24-year-old
married man and my wife has walked out on me and
our year-old son. I admit I am to blame. I used to
spend more time with my mates than with her and I
was unfaithful. But I've learnt from my mistakes and
I'd give anything to get her back as I love her so
much. Our little son cries all the time and wants his
mother. I am hoping and praying she'll come back. She
won't talk to me on the phone when I ring her
mother's place. All I want to say is that I am sorry for
hurting her so much and beg her to come back. I'd
wait for her forever if I had to, but how can I let her
know if she won't talk to me?'

'Don't give up so easily,' I wrote back. 'Write her a long letter
in which you tell her what you have told me. You can even send
her a copy of the letter you sent me and my reply to show her
that you mean what you say. Ask her to see you. Then beg her to
forgive you. If you're face-to-face it is much easier to convince
her that you love and need her and want to make a fresh start.
Tell her you are willing to set out a written 'contract' of what she
wants and what you want from the marriage and that you will
honour that contract. Above all, let her know how much you want
the three of you to be a family. There aren't many mothers who
would give up their babies, and very few wives who really want
to break up their marriage, so put all your heart in your plea.
Don't let pride prevent you from asking your friends and relatives — her mother too — to plead with her on your behalf.
Overwhelm her with love and promises which you intend to
keep. In other words, woo her all over again and no holds
barred.'

I also suggested a few sessions of counselling which would
give them greater insight into how best to resolve conflict without tearing the marriage apart. Twelve months later I was grati-
fied to receive a letter from Simon with a photo of himself and
his wife and toddler son as well as their new baby daughter. I
love stories with happy endings!

WOMEN WHO FALL FOR MARRIED MEN

In recent years there has been a new and disturbing trend — an increasing number of girls who fall in love with married men, girls who do not seem to relate to unattached, younger men. They write to me about the secret meetings, the guilt, the fear, and always the promises that come to nothing. If this happens once in a woman's life it can be put down to 'bad luck'. When it happens over and over there are more complex explanations.

The most obvious is that a woman is less afraid of commitment if a man already belongs to someone else. It is a good escape hatch if she tires of the relationship. If you are not truly committed you don't have to put as much into it and can always walk away. It is also a fact that 'somebody else's man' always seems more attractive to some women.

Yet another and far more important explanation can be traced to a woman's relationship with the first man in her life — her father. If he has been a kind and loving father who affirms and respects her, she will grow up expecting that this is how all men will treat her. If on the other hand he has been rejecting or violent towards his wife and family, she will keep on attracting men who treat her badly, and will accept that this is how things are. I have counselled women who repeatedly end up with alcoholic partners simply because they had grown up with an alcoholic father.

The dynamics of this behaviour are too complex to go into adequately here, but the theory is that when we keep tripping over the same mistake it is usually because we are trying to resolve something that went wrong and affected us deeply when we were small. We keep on repeating that same situation hoping to 'make it right' this time.

It is only by becoming aware of what the underlying problem is and dealing with it either by understanding or counselling that we come to terms with it. Karen's letter illustrates this syndrome.

'I am 28 and have had the bad luck of always falling in love with married men. I have had two unhappy experiences with men who promised me the world but wouldn't leave their wives. Now I'm in love with a married man who has three children. I met Richard

when I went to work for him. He says he'll leave his
wife and marry me when the time is right but so far
nothing has come of it. Sometimes I feel guilty but he
tells me he and his wife had drifted apart and he's
only staying because of the children. I'm confused and
don't know what to do for the best.'

This was the condensed version of Karen's long letter. She had
poured out the grief she felt when she was four and her father
left his wife for another woman. She blamed herself for years for
his going — she had not been good enough or smart enough.
She felt that if she became very ill surely he would come back,
and in fact she had a history of serious infections, but of course
he never returned.

My advice to her was to talk at a deep level with her mother
and fill in the gaps from her past. Then I urged her to see her
lover's wife and children as the people who would be affected by
her decision. It would be so much easier to dismiss them if they
were only vague, faceless people in her mind. I urged her to
forgive her father for the hurt he had caused, not so much for his
sake, but for hers. Over a period of time we corresponded and
the pieces of the jigsaw began to fall into place.

I was certain Karen kept on falling in love with married men
because she was trying to 'make right' her father's abandonment,
to find a man who would love and cherish her as he did before
he went away. She was not consciously aware of this of course,
and her perception was too narrow to realise that all the men she
fell in love with were not her father. Until she gained a broader
perspective and became aware of this she would go on repeating
the same behaviour. Not every girl who loses her father reacts in
this way. Some shake it off more easily, others develop an aversion to men and avoid any close relationships.

I did not hear from her for several months and then another
letter came. Karen was happy and buoyant.

'I have given Richard up. I thought I could never do it
but I did. I saw him with his wife and younger
daughter and realised how close they were despite his
relationship with me. For the first time I saw the real
people I was hurting (as I had been hurt) and after

that it wasn't hard to walk away. I've never felt
happier than the day I told him goodbye. Would you
believe he looked relieved that I had made the decision
for both of us? I could not have lived with myself if I
had chosen differently. As you suggested I had a real
heart-to-heart talk with my mother and now understand
many things I could not as a child. I have been
blaming her for so long. Now I've forgiven her and my
father — and myself — and I feel great.'

I like to think Karen has grown through this experience. The insights she has gained from this relationship provided valuable lessons that can be applied to future relationships. Therefore the affair with Richard was not wasted because it made her more sensitive to what she wants in a partner, and her recent experience will help her to behave from choice in the future rather than from compulsion.

The following letters, and there are many more along the same lines, could act as a warning to any girl who thinks she can win in what is nearly always a no-win situation. Stories that seem to end well are always the exception, never the rule. Consider Marion's letter:

'For six years I went out with a married man. He kept
promising he'd leave his wife but never did. Then she
left him for someone else. He was shattered and came
straight to me and we have been living together for
two years. At first I was very happy. But slowly I
began to realise I had made a terrible mistake. He is
possessive, jealous, bad-tempered, lazy and mean. He has
even hit me in a jealous rage. I'd give anything for him
to move out (we live in my unit) but I know he'd
never go. I'm so unhappy. What can I do?'

In the six years of going together, Marion's boyfriend could not have hidden the darker side of his nature all the time. There must have been clues which she refused to see. For one, a man who can treat his wife so badly for so long, without making a decision, should have alerted Marion to the fact that he had no loyalty and no integrity and that he would not treat her any better. But love, or what passes for love, is often blind.

Yet despite what she thought, she was not stuck with him forever. There was no reason to live with a man she did not love and who treated her so badly. She could order him to leave her unit although I advised her to do it in the presence of a male relative or friend who could protect her if necessary. If he was violent or threatened violence she should go to the police or a chamber magistrate or a solicitor.

'If he refuses to leave,' I said, 'wait until he goes out, then pack his belongings and leave them outside the front door, which for safety's sake, make sure is bolted. You could take extra precautions by arranging to have the lock changed.'

I agreed that all this was unpleasant and frightening, but it was not as awful as facing the rest of her life with a man with whom she could not live in peace.

Here is Michelle's letter:

'Like many of the girls who write to you, I was in love with a married man. Although I felt sorry for his wife, I just couldn't give him up. I wasn't brave enough to say the words which would have ended the relationship. He divorced his wife and we were married three months ago. He is now going out with another girl. She may be his third wife in the future. I can't blame anyone but myself. I was too blind to see what he was really like. Now I know he'll never change.'

I thanked her for sharing her sad experience. Michelle had discovered an important fact — that some men have a Casanova complex and cannot be faithful to one woman. The 'next' woman is always the one they look for. These men have no sense of worth and need to reassure themselves of their virility. They are incapable of love. He would need intensive therapy and counselling and even then there was no guarantee that he would change. I urged Michelle to try to get him to talk to her on a deeper level than he was used to, but did not hold out much hope that he would change. I suggested that she have counselling, if only for the back-up and support she needed at this time.

Claire's letter was also of the no-win variety. She wrote:

> 'I'm living with a married man who has twice left me
> to go back to his wife and then returned to me. He
> says his wife won't change so this time he says he'll
> stay with me for keeps. But I just can't be sure. Every
> time he visits his children or his wife rings up I go
> through hell. Should I trust him?'

The short answer was 'no'. I was not sure that anyone could feel secure and trusting in her position. Any man who could put his wife through such a ghastly situation could not be trusted to behave more kindly in the future with another woman. Why should he expect his wife to change when he kept leaving her? He is the one who needs to change by ending the affair. But he can't do that while Michelle is in the picture inciting him to leave his wife and family. I urged her to get out of their lives and pointed out that she would never find a partner while still involved with someone else's.

BEING RESPONSIBLE FOR YOUR OWN HAPPINESS

In the many letters I have received over the years, it is clear that most of the unhappy states that women get into are caused by allowing unhappy and pointless relationships to 'happen to them' instead of taking some action to stop them from happening. It's as if they have no say at all in their lives. This next letter is from Megan:

> 'I am 29, have been married 12 years and love my
> husband and two children. Early in 1983 I drifted into
> an affair with a man a few years younger than myself
> whom I have known and been attracted to for a few
> years. He and his family are friends of my husband
> and me. We realised it was a mistake to continue our
> sexual relationship and ceased having sex four months
> ago. I still see him often through the friendship of our
> families, a friendship we'd like to continue but which
> is being threatened by my still being attracted to him.
> This leaves me feeling terribly depressed.'

'How can you expect to get over this infatuation if you continue to set yourself up to be tested over and over again?' I asked. 'The awareness of how much you stood to lose — as well as your conscience — gave you the strength to end the affair on a physical level; you can't possibly give your emotions a chance to settle if you go on seeing him. Isn't your marriage and all it means, more important than any friendship, family or otherwise? And what about your children? Would you sacrifice their wellbeing for a passing affair? Try to avoid seeing him, make new friends and phase this one out as quickly as you can.'

Elaine wrote:

> 'After 12 years of marriage and three children, my husband has left me and is having an affair with a younger woman. He says he doesn't love me, but still wants to make love when he comes to see me. He asked me if he could come back, but I said not until he stops his affair. I love him and want him back, but will not share him with someone else.'

I applauded her decision.
'You have done the right thing in letting him know on what terms you'll have him back. For your sake it would be better to develop your life as fully as you can without him, which means, among other things, hardening your heart against his attempts to have his cake and eat it too. He has to face up to the fact that the longer he continues his affair, the less chance there is of your needing him back. Don't leave it to him to make the choices for *your* future — have the courage and the strength to make choices of your own. After all, you must consider the children's future as well.'

Although most people's sympathy would be with a betrayed wife, the 'other woman' often deserves as much compassion. Diane's story is a case in point.

> 'For the past five years I've been involved with a married man of 35 who has two children. I'm 19. He will never leave his wife — he told me straight out. I

find it hard to believe he loves me, as he says, because
I see him about once a week, if I'm lucky, and then
only for three hours as he has to rush home. I want to
finish this relationship but don't know how.'

I felt sad that Diane had given up what should have been the
carefree years of her girlhood to a furtive liaison with this man.

'You can end the unhappiness tomorrow, and open up a whole
new hopeful life for yourself, by telling this man it's over — and
sticking to your decision. Don't make any more arrangements to
meet him. Ignore any pleas or promises he may make. And
above all don't be fooled into believing that he loves you. Your
doubts on this score are valid — he doesn't. You are just a bit of
fun and spice on the side. Look around and mix with lots of
other people and make sure you crowd him out. You've been
missing an awful lot of life these past five years. Take control and
make today the beginning of the rest of your life by telling him
it's over, and stick to your resolve.'

WHEN NOT TO CONFESS

Another aspect of affairs I am often asked about is the guilt
which drives people to reveal their lapse to a spouse years after
it has happened. The writers, usually women, are full of remorse
which makes them beat down on themselves without mercy.
They would not dream of being so harsh with anyone else. This
need to 'confess' is a natural one, but as I always point out, they
would be dumping their guilt onto their unsuspecting partner
who might not be able to handle it. Nearly always, this desire to
confess is a selfish one. The need to off-load the guilty feelings
only serves to destroy the other's peace of mind. In almost every
case not telling their partner is the price they must pay for their
happiness. If they must 'confess', I urge them *not* to talk to a
relative or friend. Relatives and friends fall out sometimes and
they could never be sure their secret was safe. Debra wrote:

'Should I confess my affair and get if off my
conscience? My husband and I have been happily
married for fifteen years, but for me there has always
been a cloud over my happiness. You see, my husband

has always believed our eldest child is his. What he
doesn't know is that I had a passionate affair which
lasted only a week while I was engaged to him. We
have had four children since. But I feel I can't live
with this deceit between us any more. I am obsessed
with guilt and with the need to tell him so I can get
this weight off my conscience.'

Debra's need to clear her conscience was understandable, but
I felt that by shifting her burden onto her husband she would be
doing irreparable harm to him and their marriage and worst of
all to her eldest child. For all these years her husband has been
a father to her child in every sense of the word. Would it not be
cruel and pointless to hit him with the truth at this stage? The
truth may well be that the child is his anyway.

Yet Debra needs to get rid of her secret guilt, so I urged her to
confide in her minister or priest or rabbi, to an accredited marriage counsellor or she could ring Lifeline and 'confess' anony-
mously. That way she would resolve all her remorse without
hurting anyone. By telling her husband she would be exchang-
ing one set of regrets for another.

I must make it clear that I do not advocate deceit, but one
must weigh up all the circumstances and come up with the
choice which will create the least pain and trauma.

A heavy conscience is not the only way that guilt can be mani-
fested. Sometimes it is transferred to physical symptoms as in
the following letter from Frances.

'I have never told my husband about an affair I had
seven years before we married. We have two sons now
and a baby daughter. I'm being treated for a discharge
and I'm terrified it's an STD (sexually-transmitted
disease) resulting from that affair. Would the doctor
know? And would he keep it from me if he did?'

Of course he wouldn't keep it from her if she did have an STD
— he'd see to it that she had treatment for it. The routine tests
made before the birth of the children would have shown up any
infection then. It was clear that the past affair was preying on her

conscience and as many people do who have guilty feelings, she was punishing herself in this way. I told her that if she needed to come to terms with her conscience by talking about the past, she should see a counsellor or clergyman or a doctor. I repeated what I said at the beginning of this section — never, never, never confide such an intimate secret to a friend or relative, or the anxiety stirred up will be even more stressful than the original guilt.

Bonnie's problem was most unpleasant — blackmail always is. I tried to show her how to turn the tables on her tormentor.

> 'I'm so desperate. Last year while my husband was interstate, I had a brief affair with a man whom I happened to meet at a party. Now he threatens to tell my husband about it unless we have intercourse regularly. My husband is very possessive and I know my marriage would be at an end if he ever found out. I've pleaded with this man to go away and leave me alone for my children's sakes but he just laughs at me. I know he is going to tell my husband and I also know the results will be drastic.'

'No more drastic, I assure you, than the results of being blackmailed into a form of prostitution by this wretched man,' I answered. 'Call his bluff and stop seeing him. It's most unlikely he'll go to your husband, for this would reveal his own part in the plan, which might enrage your husband. If, on the other hand, he does talk to your husband, it's his word against yours and I'd advise you to deny everything and say he is being revengeful because you have rejected his advances. He has scared you enough for your foolishness.'

7

Being Single in the 90s

IN OUR PRESENT WORLD, our attitudes to life and sex are so much more relaxed and so many of the old restraints have been discarded that we might be forgiven for believing that single people today have it made. The letters I receive tell me this is not so. What I hear is that young people have never been more isolated than in this age of easy relationships.

Twenty-one years ago I had letters from young teenagers asking me for an itemised 'recipe' on how to attract a boy. Now I receive many letters from young readers and an increasing number from women — and men — in their thirties who despair of ever meeting a compatible partner. It's as if the new freedom has brought new expectations and made them self-conscious with the opposite sex. It has also made them more suspicious and sometimes cynical. What is surprising is that there are fewer and fewer places where men and women have a chance to meet. Clubs and bars have been dubbed 'meat markets' and are shunned by many. Meeting through personal columns in newspapers, on radio programmes and through introduction agencies is acceptable to some, and there are even courses on 'dating and mating'.

The Women's Movement has made some men wary of women and afraid of commitment, and women's expectations of what they want in a man are sometimes intimidating. But underneath all that, both sexes want and need each other desperately. Getting together is the problem.

Mostly women write of being too tall, too short, overweight, not pretty enough, too quiet, too talkative, or too depressed. I've heard them all. And even as I tell them that men are not looking for perfection, I know it is their own self-doubts which are keeping them from meeting partners.

Men's letters tell the same story — that they are lonely and confused and longing for companionship. If anything, men are more vulnerable in love than women. They are unsure of themselves and are looking for warmth and acceptance, for someone to love them. They cover up their need with a show of bravado — the very thing which turns women away for fear they will be rejected. Women have the advantage in that we can talk about our feelings to other women and gain their support and a certain relief. A man's ego prevents him from doing this with his mates and he suffers in silence.

I'M TOO SHY

Shyness is one of the most common problems.

> 'I'm not usually a shy person, but around guys who
> are good-looking or guys I like, I just can't talk. I've
> just started a new job and because of this problem I
> can't socialise. I'm scared I'll say something really
> stupid and they will think I *am* stupid and reject me.
> Please suggest an answer. Thank you for your time.'

This was my answer: 'The shyness you describe is a common complaint for both sexes. Men have often written to me about being too shy to approach an attractive woman. You don't have to do anything much to be part of a group, you know. You can stay with your quietness and it will pass if you don't make a big deal out of it. You are taking yourself too seriously over something which you will eventually grow out of if you treat it lightly. The way to handle it is to look interested when in a group and show you are listening. That will make you just as much a part of the conversation as those who do all the talking. Listeners are always in such short supply! And remember that others will take you at your own evaluation. If you know you are not stupid, and respect yourself in a quiet way, others will get the message and treat you with the same respect.'

And now a letter from the other side of the fence:

'I am a 17-year-old boy and have a problem: I am self-conscious. The main disadvantage with this is that it stops me from mixing with girls. I have never had a girlfriend in my life and get very depressed and angry when I see guys my age with girlfriends. There is one girl I've really liked for the past year but have always been shy of her as she is so popular. She has been very helpful with schoolwork and is always friendly to me but when I try to talk to her my mouth dries up and I feel a fool. After a while she didn't talk to me much any more and I feel I have hurt her feelings. I've wanted to ring her at times but I'm too shy to do even that. I am sick of being this way as it stops me from doing the things I want to do. How can I overcome this?'

'Now that you have become aware of how shyness can wreck your life and stop you from doing what you really want to do, you are more readily motivated to change. It might help you to know that many famous people, some of whom are constantly in the pubic eye, have had to overcome self-consciousness in order to succeed. You are right about this girl being hurt by your behaviour. Shy people often give the impression they are snobs, and she is probably avoiding you because she thinks you are rejecting her. Silly isn't it? Why not follow your natural feelings and ask her out? And when you know her just a little better, why not admit that you are shy? She will welcome your honesty and may admit her own vulnerability.

Don't be put off if you are occasionally rejected. We all have our share of rejections, but at least there is the possibility of success, whereas doing nothing is certain to bring you nothing. Relating easily to other people gets easier and easier with practice, so start practising.'

HOW DO I MEET PEOPLE?

Michael's letter was only one of many I receive with the same problem: 'Where do you meet nice women?'

'I am a male, going on 25 and am slightly confused and alone. I am told I have average build and looks, I go to all the places where you're supposed to meet young ladies, such as clubs and bars, but they are either too young or looking for husbands. It has also been my experience that guys are not the only ones with one-track minds. Where are the decent girls these days? Could the fact that I am in the Armed Forces have anything to do with it? Are girls impressed by the uniform or by the security?'

'You are not alone, young man — many guys not in the Forces have similar problems,' I replied. 'All I can say is that perhaps the places where you go are the wrong places for serious-minded men to meet nice girls who don't have one-track minds. Of course, you can't blame them for doing exactly what you're doing and that is looking for a partner of the opposite sex. There are plenty of decent girls around, I assure you, but you do not find them in pick-up places — you're more likely to meet them in a club where the members are actually doing something together, such as participating in sport, or taking classes or courses of interest to them. You can find out what is available by contacting your local community centre. The enthusiasm generated in such groups who are doing something for others and enjoying themselves at the same time, is the best friendship-maker in the world for both sexes.

'The thing is to keep trying and not give up after a failure or two. Decent women are just as keen to meet decent men, and I have many letters to prove it. Keep trying and believing that it will happen and it will.'

In the last few years I have received more and more letters like this next one from Kathryn.

'I am a 33-year-old woman and although I have an excellent job and many friends, I feel my life is a failure. I am told I am attractive, dress well and have good values, but I can't seem to meet a man who wants a long-term relationship. I have been out with three men in the past three years who only wanted to

have a good time and nothing more. They backed-off
after a few months. I see some of my schoolfriends
with good marriages and children and some who are
not so happy and it makes me very cautious about the
kind of man I would welcome into my life. Sometimes I
feel that I'll end up a lonely, miserable old lady and it
scares me. Lately I've been depressed and unhappy and
life doesn't seem worth living. How do I meet a man I
can love and who will love me?'

My answer had to be frank, and so I replied. 'Maybe you're not
going to meet such a man, but that doesn't mean you have to
crawl into a hole. You are looking at only one solution and have
an idealised idea of what you're missing out on, without giving a
thought to the positive steps you can take to make a full, happy
life as a single woman.

'As you are noting in your friends' lives, marriage is no guarantee of happiness. No one can make you happy, not marital
status, not money or success — nothing except yourself and the
way you invest your energy and intelligence into turning your
life into what you want. You seem to attract your share of men
and that is understandable since you are attractive and successful
and healthy male achievers are drawn to women who match
their own get up and go. Perhaps you are over-cautious and this
comes across as aloofness which makes them get in first to save
face. Or your expectations may be too rigid. Perhaps you need to
compromise a little and give men a chance. They may possess
qualities which are not evident in the first few meetings.

'I suggest that you give up the waiting game and invest in
being more involved in the world around you, increase your
circle of friends and acquaintances and the areas of interest that
fill your life. Above all, be good to yourself in every way you can
think of. You are the best friend you will ever have. Once you
make peace with your singleness and accept that you may never
have a permanent, loving commitment, you will prove you are
taking charge of your life and are more likely to meet the man
you could love and who could love you.'

Here is Jill's letter:

'I am a 20-year-old university student. My problem is

that I am not satisfied with my life. It is incomplete
and I feel that something is missing. I am an average-
looking person and feel that I have a good personality,
however I do not seem to attract the opposite sex. They
do not seem to be interested in me at all. They turn
away when I show I am interested in them and I feel I
can never get close to a boy or even talk to one. I
know I am not trying too hard. My friends do not have
this problem and I am feeling lonely, confused and
desperate. I would love to marry and have children in
the not-too-distant future but somehow I can't see this
happening. Will it be like this for the rest of my life?'

Apart from her name, she signed her letter 'Concerned Reject'
which told me she had written herself off. It was no wonder
everyone else seemed to have written her off too. Part of her
problem was that she was concentrating on what was missing
from her life rather than on what she already has. This attitude
can come across as gloomy whingeing which can be embarrass-
ing and is very off-putting. It was clear she had very low self-
esteem and that no one was going to treat her any better than
she treats herself.

'If I were you,' I wrote, 'I'd ask a good and trusted friend to
give it to me between the eyes and tell me if I have any manner-
ism or trait which puts people off. We all do or say things of
which we are not aware.'

I pointed out that at 20 she was hardly over the hill. It would
be in her best interests to develop her potential and her life and
not be in such a hurry to become involved with a boyfriend
before she knows what she really wants. It is while she is busy
living and learning and enjoying it that she will meet up with
like-minded people and will be more likely to find that 'special
person'.

Claire's letter expressed what many women feel — that men are
after only one thing, sex.

'I am 24 and very unhappy. You see, I've never had a
boyfriend although I try to be pleasant and go to all

the places where you're supposed to meet men. I play
tennis, and belong to a social club, but the men are
either too young or after one thing — sex. I'm not the
type to jump into bed with a boy the first time I go
out with him, so I'm not very popular. Don't boys like
a decent girl any more? Is sex all they want? How does
a girl get to meet a decent guy these days? If you go
anywhere by yourself, the men think you're an easy
pick-up and all they want is a one-night stand.'

I had to tell Claire that sex was not what all men wanted,
unless a woman shows either subtly or otherwise, that it's all she
has to offer or withhold. What about tenderness, enthusiasm,
sharing simple pleasures, understanding and ordinary everyday
cheerfulness? These are basic human needs, alongside the
sexual one, and most men look for these qualities. Men who are
only after sex have no respect for themselves or for a woman. I
urged Claire to try to acquire some confidence in herself and, to
continue to go out with friends of both sexes.

'Gradually you'll feel that, like everyone else, you are accepted
as a friend and a worthwhile human being. Love and romance
will eventually develop, but not while that is all you look for in
your relationships with men.'

'As for meeting men, the place to meet them is anywhere and
everywhere. Consider these possibilities: the supermarket, the
laundromat, furniture stores, menswear stores, airports, auctions,
restaurants, bars, lunch-counters, university libraries, university
bookstores, art galleries, church, social clubs, evening classes
(photography is supposed to be a good class to meet men!),
political groups, environmental groups, golf tournaments, hard-
ware stores, boat and automobile shows, martial arts classes,
dancing classes . . .

'The list is almost endless and you can add your own ideas.
And don't knock back your friends' or family's attempts to match
you up with a brother or cousin of theirs. All they are doing is
making it possible for two young people to meet. After that it's
up to you. The deciding factor, though, is your attitude to others
and above all to yourself. You must believe in people and like
them, and you must believe in yourself and your ability to attract
the man you would like, before it can happen.'

Sara's letter was very revealing. She wrote:

> 'I am an attractive 40-year-old, recently divorced, no children, and comfortably off. My problem? I'm looking for a man, and believe me, it isn't easy to find the right one. Most men of forty plus are married, and if they're not, I'm not interested because it means they're either homosexuals, selfish, or too set in their ways. I love life too much to go through the rest of it alone, but where do I start looking?'

'I'd say you start by looking at yourself, your prejudices and very closed mind,' I replied. 'Has it ever occurred to you that many of the men who are over forty and have never married, may never have met the girl they wanted to marry and who wanted to marry *them*? Just because they live alone doesn't mean they are necessarily selfish. We all become set in our ways if we only have ourselves to please. This, of course, also applies to many women who have never married. Don't dismiss the men you meet so readily, or *you* could be accused of being set in your ways.'

YOUR HEART'S ON YOUR SLEEVE

We must all learn to protect ourselves. Marylin wrote:

> 'I'm a very emotional girl who falls in love with every guy I meet. It's great while it lasts — but that is usually only about a few weeks because the boys in question seem to be more shallow than I am and back off. I don't hear from them again and soon find out they are going with someone else. I'd love to meet a nice guy and have a steady relationship but somehow I never succeed. All that happens is that I get hurt again and again. I'm fed up. What can I do?'

'You are always looking to be in love because you have a great empty gap in your emotional life — a deficit — which you are compulsively trying to fill. Because you are lacking in self-esteem, you feel you are unworthy of being loved and are so convinced of this at a deep level, that you only attract men who are shallow and uncaring. You deserve a steady man who appreciates you and you need to believe this with all your heart. Of course, you must be prepared to work on a relationship, to accept trust and respect and return them in full measure. But the first step is to love and nurture that needy part of yourself.

'Talk gently to that deprived child inside you and let her know she is loved and cherished by you. Write down a list of all the things you like and admire about yourself. This is not being immodest — it is an acknowledgement of your being. Add to the list each day or as you think of something positive about yourself. You'll be surprised at how much you will find to admire. Then relax and be patient. It's your desperation which forces you to make quick, unstable choices. Take it slowly.'

YOU CAN SET THE PACE

Susie wrote:

> 'I'm 19. I've been out with a few men but I always
> freeze up if they touch me, and I can't bear to be
> kissed. I only want friendship with a man at present,
> but they all seem to expect more. When I see how
> relaxed and uninhibited my friends are with men, I
> think there must be something wrong with me.'

Why do women feel there is something wrong with them because they want to be touched and kissed only by men with whom they feel warm and friendly?

'It's clear that so far you have not felt this way about any of the men you have been out with. You need to come to terms with the fact that most men who take you out are going to make some kind of physical approach, if only to find out what your views are, and also because they may feel that you would think less of them if they didn't. So you need to tone down the freezing treatment and just tell them how you feel about touching. Then you will have a better chance of achieving a friendship at your pace — a pace which suits more men than you realise.'

WHAT DO WOMEN WANT?

Men do not write to me nearly as often as women about their loneliness. Perhaps they regard such an admission as a sign of weakness. But I have had some touching letters from them and whenever I have published such a letter in my page, the mail from women wanting to make contact is overwhelming.

Peter's letter was open and honest and it was clear he wanted an honest answer.

'I hope you can help me sort out this problem. I'm totally confused where girls are concerned. I've had several girlfriends during the past two years — nothing serious, just to go around with — but I do not seem to hit it off with any of them. If I try to be a 'gentleman' and ask them for a kiss, they nearly always say 'no' and then make fun of me with their friends. If I just kiss them without warning, I may get a kiss, but they get all outraged and angry and the evening is spoilt. Don't think I'm just after sex because I'm not. I like the girls I go out with and have respect for them, but they confuse me so much I just don't know how to act. Can you give me a few guidelines and put me on the right track? I'm 17.'

I was happy to reassure him.

'You'd like to be smooth and suave in your dealings with girls but that takes years to achieve and is not possible at your age. Both you and they are beginners, still finding out what's what, and quite naturally, getting a few crossed wires. This doesn't mean you're a failure or a bungler — it's life. And don't try to shift your technique from one extreme to the other as you seem to be doing at present. You must be yourself and act naturally without being an old-world hero or a cave-dweller. Then you'll gradually sort out the girls who like you just as you are — and you can't please them all.

'One last bit of advice: Don't react so dramatically to their behaviour, whether they appear to make fun when you ask for a kiss or get angry when you grab one. Both these are well-known face-saving devices for girls who may want to be kissed, but don't want to appear all that eager.'

Mark's letter was unusual and raised some interesting points.

> 'May I use your column to ask one question of your
> women readers?' he wrote. 'Do they know how hurtful
> and dishonest it is to play hard to get? I'm a bachelor
> of 35 and women I find attractive and want to get
> involved with are always trotting out the old line:
> "Let's be friends and see what happens". Rather than
> making me more keen, it makes these women a waste
> of time. Why do they do it?'

I had to inform him that playing hard to get has pretty well
died out. Men and women are now much more honest.

'So, you are faced with one of two answers. Firstly, the women
you meet don't find you attractive and don't want to get involved,
or secondly, your let's-pitch-straight-in attitude puts them off.
You don't appear to consider women as individuals. So it's your
approach and your attitude which is letting you down.'

I pointed out that I saw nothing offensive in a woman wanting
to begin with friendship before becoming too involved. Women
are more discerning — and wary — these days, and in any case,
being good friends is the best beginning for any relationship.

Jim's letter was about a different problem yet a similar effect.

> 'I'm 22 and just don't seem able to keep a girlfriend. I
> attract them easily enough, but they find excuses after
> going out two or three times. My last girlfriend even
> got angry and told me I'm too intense and possessive,
> and that I scared her. I've always thought girls liked to
> feel admired and to be made a fuss of. What's wrong?'

'Some girls like to be treated in this way and some don't,' I
answered. 'What you seem to be doing wrong is trying too hard
and treating all girls the same instead of as individuals, and even
with girls who like to be made a fuss of all the time, you seem to
be overdoing it a bit. So give up any general beliefs about what
girls like and just take your cues from the girl you're with. Good
luck next time!'

WHY DO I CHOOSE BAD MEN?

Debbie expressed a problem in her letter which crops up often.

> 'I am a 17-year-old female and for some reason I seem
> to be attracted to men who don't express great interest
> in me or who don't treat me very well. Once someone
> starts really liking me I lose interest in them. I don't
> have much confidence, so you'd think it would be
> normal for me to want a perfect gentleman who opens
> doors for you and treats you like a lady. I've been out
> occasionally with that type but they do nothing for me.
> Do you think I should see a psychiatrist?'

It was clear to me the problem was more complex than she knew.

'There are many possible reasons why you behave as you do. Look back on how things were in your family, especially with your father. Did he give you the love and support one expects from a loving father, or was he off-hand and rejecting of you? A girl's father is the first model on whom she bases her expectations of men in her life.

'It is also possible your low self-esteem leads you to believe you don't deserve to be treated well. You then unconsciously choose men who will confirm this by treating you badly. Or you could be feeling guilty about something you did or failed to do, and you punish yourself through the ill-treatment you know you'll get from these men.

'For whatever reason, this has now become a pattern and you can't help yourself. You are driven to act as you do. You need a counsellor, not necessarily a psychiatrist. A psychologist with whom you feel comfortable would be a good person to start with. Enquire at your Community Health Centre and learn how to break this destructive pattern before you destroy your life.'

IS A DIVORCEE A BAD RISK?

Magda wrote:

> 'Ever since my divorce a year ago I have been keen to
> find the right man so I can remarry. I'm not really the

sort to be without a man in my life and my son needs a father. But although I meet a lot of men, I don't seem to attract them any more. I had a terrific boyfriend while the divorce was going through — we were very much in love — but even he lost interest after three months.

'I'm beginning to wonder if a broken marriage makes a woman a bad risk or something. All the men I meet seem to want a casual affair. They become visibly cool when it's obvious that I want more than this. I'm only 27 and getting very lonely and depressed.'

I tried to give Magda another viewpoint on her problem. 'Divorce is a big change in your life and you need to change with it. By saying 'I'm not the sort to do this or that', you are more likely to stay exactly as you are and not change, which means you will limit your life and remain stuck with all your old problems and attitudes.

'One change you could make is to consider how rich and worthwhile your life and your son's can be right now. As long as you feel you need the love of another adult to survive, all your relationships will be geared towards having someone rescue you. That puts a big responsibility on a man for a start.

'If you're continually turning down casual affairs, there's obviously no doubt about you being attractive to men. In time you'll find someone who, like you, is looking for something serious. But this is more likely to happen when a man is no longer a "must", but someone with whom you can share a life already made full by you alone.'

CAN I ASK A BOY OUT?

Karla's letter read like something I would have received in the 70s, yet it only came the other day. She wrote:

'I have been invited to a dinner-dance soon to which all my friends are going, and taking partners. I am 19 and don't have a steady so I won't be able to go. I'm interested in a boy at work whom I'd like to ask, but I'm so afraid he'd refuse, although friends tell me he's

interested in me. Even in these days of 'equality' I've
seen boys shy off when a girl asks them out so I'm
scared of making a fool of myself. But I want to go to
the dinner-dance.'

'Have you heard the saying: "Nothing ventured, nothing
gained"?' I asked. 'Living involves risks, and you've really
nothing to lose by asking this boy. I can't promise that he'll
accept — he may loathe dinner-dances. But it sounds to me as if
he'll say "yes". If he refuses, well, we all get let-downs in our
lifetime and if we avoid facing them, we avoid living. Go ahead
and ask him, and if he refuses, ask someone else — maybe a
relative or a friend's brother — to go with you'.

IT'S BEST TO BE HONEST

'Recently I met a terrific girl on a plane trip interstate.
I didn't think I'd ever see her again so I had a great
time putting myself across as a successful, much-
travelled, social man-about-town, none of which is true.
I am 35, personable and sincere, and reasonably
successful in my career, but nowhere as exciting as I
made out to this girl. At the end of the journey we'd
got on so well, we swapped phone numbers. I'd love to
see her again but I don't dare because of those lies.'

I did my best to reassure him.
'You're not the only young man to add some extra colour and
excitement to your image. Most women know this, but are pretty
sensitive to a man's pride and wouldn't say outright that they'd
taken all your stories with a pinch of salt. So, if you do get in
touch with one another, make only a passing reference to the
fairy stories you told her.'

8

What About Sex?

IN 1970 WHEN my column first appeared, the sexual revolution was only just beginning to make itself felt. People were embarrassed about problems related to sex, and tippy-toed around them, trying to disguise what was really troubling them.

In those days virginity was still regarded as the ideal until marriage and I received hundreds of letters from young people asking me on a scale of one to ten how far you could go in petting and still be regarded as a virgin. That was the question most often asked by teenagers of that time. In the mid-to-late seventies there was a flurry of letters begging me to give them the name of a doctor who could restore their virginity. Girls who were about to be married did not want their future husband to find out about their past. I could only advise them that a semblance of virginity could be restored and suggested they talk to their doctor who would refer them to an expert.

In the late seventies and eighties loss of virginity no longer rated as a problem and the letters on petting dropped off completely. I guessed that many girls were going to the top of the scale without preamble. The sexual revolution was already peaking and I was receiving letters from girls who considered it a reason for shame that they were virgins at 18 and even younger. Girls were bragging to their girlfriends about their sexual exploits which were clearly non-existent. Some even wrote to me about the white lies they told in this regard so as to appear to be keeping up with their friends. Many girls at this time gained a reputation simply through their tall tales and not their actions.

This made many less confident girls feel as though they were excluded and not conforming to the expectations of the group. Many jumped in feet first, not because they wanted to, but because they thought they ought to and found themselves out of their depth when it was too late.

In the seventies I was appalled by the number of letters from men who wanted to indulge in wife-swapping. They were the heady days when people behaved as though sex had just been discovered. Many, who did not know how to deal with this newfound freedom, lost all sense of proportion and went wild. This was the time when total freedom was the ultimate goal. The motto of those years was 'Let it all hang out'. They had never heard that the flip side of freedom is responsibility.

Older people wanted to make up for the restrictions in their own youth and followed the young in their mindless conduct, abdicating their role as parents and becoming even more confused than their offspring. The stable environment of family life was no longer there for kids to come home to.

In the mid-seventies I remember mentioning the word 'orgasm' in my column. I believe I was the first columnist to do so in a magazine and I was flooded with letters from women, some of whom had been happily married for 30 years or more and had never experienced an orgasm and who now wanted one. At the time I wondered if I had opened a Pandora's box of troubles by letting them know what they had missed instead of allowing them to enjoy the rewards of closeness which had kept them happy so far.

These were the years when we became self-indulgent and assumed it was okay to do our own thing when we felt like it, regardless of the consequences to ourselves or anyone else. This often set into action a mindless sequence of events which ended in unwanted pregnancies, unwise marriages, disease and social problems. We seemed to be hell-bent on self-destruction.

From the late eighties the pendulum began to swing back, slowly at first, and now I notice signs that it is gaining momentum. People seem to be interested with more basic concerns such as relationships, commitments and what is best for their children and their future. Thinking of the future and the environment has had a sobering effect on most people. Today we are more aware of other people and their needs, and universal love is spoken of more freely as a healing force. It's as if hard times have made us pull together. AIDS has halted the sexual revolution in its tracks. Where celibacy was once regarded as something to be ridiculed, it is now being considered as a viable alternative.

BRAGGING ABOUT SEX

'I'm 17. The other day I was talking with some friends and they asked if I'd ever had sex. When I replied honestly that I hadn't, they looked surprised and burst out laughing. Am I wrong to refuse my steady boyfriend whom I like a lot? Since that day I've felt like a freak.'

'Well, you're not a freak,' I replied, 'and you'd better believe it. Your friends, like most teenagers in a crowd, were trying to imply they were all sexually experienced and that you were not. You'd be crazy to take this universal form of one-upmanship as a guideline either to their behaviour or yours. Sexual relations have nothing to do with what anyone else does or believes is right — it's what you believe that matters. You obviously don't think sex with your boyfriend would be right. So that's it.'

Craig wrote:

'I'm a 20-year-old man and have had a lot of sexual experience. My present girlfriend is 18 and a virgin. She says she wants to stay that way until she's married. But my past has taught me that most girls who say "no" are really hoping that the man will be masterful and pressure them into lovemaking. Am I right?'

'You would be right,' I said, 'if you were living in a fantasy world but as far as facts are concerned, you are absolutely wrong. Your own fantasy of women wanting to be taken by force is appallingly selfish and can be frightening and damaging for the woman involved. Even if you take a lot of time and gentle persuasion for your seduction with your current girlfriend, and guard against making her pregnant, it's still totally wrong because it ignores the rational choice she has made. She has to answer "yes" of her own free will before you can contemplate making love.'

SHE SAID I WAS IMPOTENT

Boys don't often write in with their sex problems — they are more sensitive about this subject than girls — but I get the occasional letter. Here is one from Ron:

> "There's a girl I really liked but couldn't get near her for a while. She was very popular with other boys but eventually she agreed to go out with me. After we'd been going out for a few weeks we went to bed, I might add at her suggestion. To my horror, I was unable to make love to her. She laughed at me and told me to grow up, and said it meant I was impotent. We haven't met since. I'm 20 and feel my life is over. Where can I go for help?"

I replied: 'You were just plain unlucky to be dazzled by a girl who is cruel and silly — a sad combination. Impotence means a failure to get an erection over a long period of time, when there's no obvious reason for failure. It's not an isolated failure to make love, especially when there are several real reasons for it — like the first attempt with a particular girl you thought out of reach and special, your lack of confidence and her unsympathetic reaction to this lack. So look on this as an isolated failure that can happen to anyone and often does. The only "help" you need is another more loving relationship with a more sensitive girl.'

I DON'T ENJOY SEX

Nicole wrote:

> 'I am 16 and my boyfriend is 18. We have been having sex for the past two months but have been going steady for eight months. The problem is I don't enjoy sex. Should I or am I too young, or is there something

wrong with me? He wants me to go on the Pill but I
don't trust it. I also feel guilty because I'm not a
virgin. My close friends are virgins and they sort of
say sex is dirty. Is it?'

I replied, 'No, there is nothing wrong with you, and yes, you
are too young. Not that there is any age for enjoying sex, but it is
an adult activity, and if you are not emotionally ready for it and if
it goes against your own deeply-felt beliefs and values, then you
will feel guilty and uncomfortable as you have found out.

'Sex is not dirty (how can the very act of creation be dirty?),
but when we misuse it by flouting, not so much the prevailing
social customs but our own convictions, it becomes a destructive
rather than a positive force. Don't be pushed into going on the
Pill (although I trust you are taking precautions against pregnancy and sexually-transmitted diseases) or into having sex if
you don't want to. It's your right to say "no" just as it's your right
to say "yes" when you're older and meet someone to whom you
can feel committed.'

Nell wrote:

'I am 18 years of age and have been having regular
intercourse for four years. The problem is that I don't
enjoy it as much as I'd like to. That is, I've never
climaxed during intercourse, only when I masturbate.
At first I thought it might be the fault of the guy I
was with, but I have slept with many different men,
nearly all one-night stands, and all with the same
result. My friends say I'm getting a bad reputation
because I enjoy going out, seducing a man, sleeping
with him and then looking for another. Maybe I'm
looking for the satisfaction I need, or is there
something wrong with me mentally or physically
because I need to sleep with different men every few
days and never climax?'

I did not intend to sound 'preachy' but I had to tell her the
truth as I saw it.

'What you're looking for is not satisfaction but love and physical closeness, the kind we all need but don't always get in our

childhood years. Some people's needs are so great that they always feel they missed out as children, and as adults they are forever trying to fill what seems a bottomless well by behaving in all kinds of destructive ways, including promiscuously. Each time you seduce another man you hope to find this closeness, but of course you don't because you're looking in the wrong place.

'Begin by loving and nurturing yourself — it won't come from anywhere else unless you can do this. I know from my years as counsellor that this is easier in theory than in practice, so I urge you to seek the help of a professional counsellor at your community health centre. It will be easier for you if you have ongoing support and back-up.'

I FEEL USED

Many girls, like Gina, write about feeling 'used':

'I'm rapt in this boy and have been going with him for nearly eight months,' she wrote. 'The only trouble is he doesn't seem to care about me the same way I do about him. He seems to want to see me only when he wants sex and that's all. I feel very much used but I always say "yes" rather than not see him at all.'

'You say "yes" against your better judgment only because you think too little of yourself,' I replied. 'You seem to have the idea that his callous treatment is all you deserve and it's better than not having a boyfriend at all. But it will lower your self-esteem more and more the longer it goes on. Without him you'd get back the feeling of being worthy of someone's real affection and admiration. And you'd find that someone before long. While he's around, sapping your confidence and self-respect, you'll never give yourself the chance to meet anyone more worthwhile.'

The next letter from Lisa again concerns one of the most basic needs we humans have — the need to be held and cared about and not necessarily in a sexual way.

'You must help me before I make a complete mess of my life. I have never been very popular with guys so

when one shows an interest in me, I do anything to
keep him. By that I mean I let them have sex with me.
I know it's wrong and I feel cheap afterwards because I
know I had no true feelings for them. After that they
drop me and don't want to see me any more. I don't
know why I do it — all I want is for someone to hold
me and care for me. Do you think there's something
wrong with me?'

I was pleased to reassure her on at least one point.

'There's nothing wrong with you,' I replied. 'You have the
same human need we all have, to be cared about and touched
and held. The mistake you are making is in believing that this
need is only sexual. It isn't. What you are searching for is a deep
affection and caring and you give anything and everything in the
hope of finding it. As you have found out, it doesn't work. Until
you care about yourself and believe you are worth something, no
one else will believe it.

'Why not get in touch with a Community Health Centre near
you and ask about self-development courses or assertiveness
training courses? By meeting other young, like-minded people
and finding out what makes you tick, you will gain self-esteem
and make new friendships where the focus is on sharing and
caring and not only on sex. Don't sell yourself so short.'

I WON'T HAVE SEX

The next letter from Julie is typical of many I receive each week.

'I am sure my problem is shared by many girls my age.
I am 17 and have a nice boyfriend. We have known
each other for a couple of months and although I love
him very much and he says he loves me, I'm afraid I'll
lose him as soon as he finds out I won't have sex with
him. He doesn't continually pressure me to go to bed
with him but sometimes when we are alone he suggests
it and I always refuse. He doesn't seem to be really
mad when I say no, and he hasn't said he'll drop me if
I don't, but I'm just worried that he might start
looking round for other girls who are more ready to

oblige. I've tried explaining that I have to be sure, but
I don't think he understands. What can I tell him that
will make him understand?'

'There are a few things you need to understand,' I answered.
'Despite their randy reputation, not all boys want you "for one
thing only" as so many girls seem to think. There are still lots of
boys who relate to girls as human beings first and want to get to
know and enjoy their company before a more intimate commitment is even mentioned. But you must also be aware that a boy's
sexual urge is more urgent than a girl's and more tied in with his
idea of himself as a man. Therefore he may feel that he ought to
ask you for sex in case you think less of him if he doesn't. He
may even have been relieved when you declined! Relax and be
warm, cheerful, understanding and fun-to-be-with and continue
to say no, if that is how you feel. If you say it lovingly and gently,
he won't drop you. Girls who are ready to "oblige" are more
readily dropped, I assure you.'

I'M STILL A VIRGIN

This next letter from Maree is unusual, but it touches on many
issues which are relevant in this section.

'I'm 31 and still a virgin. I'm surrounded at work and
in my day-to-day life by younger people who seem to be
sexually experienced, married or not. Because of this,
I'm ashamed to say I think of little else except sex. I
live alone and hardly have any social life so my
fantasies are all that keep me going — but they are
driving me crazy. I am obsessed with having sex but
how can I do this without losing my peace of mind?
My letter has probably shocked you, but I desperately
need your advice.'

I was not shocked by Maree's need to have sex since it is a
natural craving.

'Where you are a little off beam is in your assumption that it is
merely a physical need that can be fulfilled in an impersonal
way. Even more important is the need to make warm, intimate

contact with another person who is congenial and loving. Remember, though it's fashionable to deny it, both men and women hope for a degree of security and simple, kindly comforting in their sex lives. What you must understand is that you can't have a sex life without any other kind of life. While you sit at home alone thinking about sex, there's not the slightest chance of your ever being loved and wanted. Only by getting out and mixing with people will you discover that everyone else is not blissfully fulfilled sexually and emotionally. There are many, many people like you, longing for friendship, love and sex.'

Sharon's letter illustrates another aspect of virginity in this modern age:

'At the age of 20 I'm still a virgin. I've had my fair share of offers but have always believed that it's something special and that one should think carefully about whom you choose to sleep with. Now, since I'm the only virgin I know, I've begun to wonder if my views are wrong. However, my main problem is that I seem to be afraid of sex. Who I choose means so much to me that I'm afraid to make a commitment in case I make a mistake. I've now met a man I'm attracted to, but I'm scared of his advances and the inevitable results. I've thought of going on the Pill, but I'm afraid it might make me like some of my friends who take sex as a daily event with anyone who happens to be there at the time. I don't know why I think like this as I've been brought up to know that sex is natural and nothing to be ashamed of. My parents had no inhibitions. I have a good relationship with them and have long talks with my mum, but it doesn't help. Should I discuss this with my boyfriend?'

'What you're afraid of is not sex but indiscriminate sex. Surrounded as you are by people whose values are different from yours, you have become uncertain and confused, fearful of making a mistake you'd regret very deeply. However, this also prevents you from relating to boys even on a friendly level for fear of what might happen, and so deprives you of many poten-tial rewards. How will you ever know who is the right man if you never get close enough to find out? In fact, this attitude is more likely to lead to a bad choice.

'Talk about your feelings with this young man — then he might tell you how he feels and you'll be on the way to really knowing each other. Then trust yourself.'

POSITIVE AIDS TEST

Leanne's letter made me reflect for a long time on the sort of world we have now and are handing over to our children.

> 'I am 14 and have been having sex with my boyfriend for about two years now. He has had an AIDS test and it was positive. I don't want to tell my parents so what do I do?'

It was a difficult problem to answer.

'You may have been one of the lucky ones and have not been affected but that doesn't mean you'll be lucky forever. I strongly advise you to go to one of the walk-in clinics which exist in every state or go to a medical practitioner and ask for a blood test. If you are free of the virus, don't push your luck. Don't have sex until you are old enough to be responsible about it. And don't be misled by any boy even if he appears clean-cut and 'clear'. Remember the words of the AIDS Council's advertising cam-paign — "When you have sex with someone, you don't have sex with only that person, but with all their past sexual partners before you." Don't think it can't happen to you. It can. And see if you can find the right time to talk to your parents about these things. At your tender age you need loving guidance. Talk to them.'

DEMANDING LOVERS

> 'Although I'm very much in love with my 22-year-old boyfriend, I'm really frightened by his continual demands to have sex. He says it will deepen our relationship. (He also assures me that he'll take

'precautions.) But I'm so afraid he'll turn nasty if I
don't satisfy him or please him. He already gets angry
if I don't let him handle me as much as he wants. I'm
16. I am sick with worry about losing him but it
seems that this could happen even if I do give in to
his demands, as well as if I don't give in.'

My answer is frank. 'Deep down you already know you're boxed-in, and that no matter what you do it's not going to make you happy for long. Be brave and face the situation as it is and not how you wish it were or how you think it might be if you did this or that. First, drop the assumption that there must be a way to make this relationship come right. Ask yourself if it's worth keeping on with it at all. What would be deepened if you slept together whenever he wanted to is what there already is in your relationship — your fear of him, his selfishness and exploitation of you, his anger when things don't go his way, and your anxiety about being rejected.

'The fact is that he sees you as an object with no wishes or feelings of your own and your friendship can never come right unless he begins to see you as a person instead. This change sounds unlikely — he is obviously far too selfish — but perhaps you could at least talk to him about it. But in the final analysis, it's your fear of him that really shows the relationship isn't right.You can never be happy outside a warm climate of real loving.'

This next letter from Carol arrived not so long ago and I include it here because even after so many years of reading unusual letters, it disturbed me.

'I am 16 years old and recently my boyfriend told me
that he wanted us to participate in group sex with
some of his friends. I have never done anything like
this before and would feel uncomfortable doing so, but
I do not want to lose him over this. He says it would
spice up our relationship and bring us closer together,
but I don't see this as being true. Do you think I
should give it a go? Is there anything wrong with
group sex? Please advise me.'

It took a great effort not to tell her what I thought of this boy, but I told her what I thought of his suggestion.

'That small voice inside you is telling you what to do and what not to do, so listen to it. Since there is no such thing as 100% safe sex, what your boyfriend is asking you to do could expose you to sexually-transmitted disease or pregnancy. But apart from these very real risks, this act would destroy your self-respect and peace of mind. If you allow yourself to be blackmailed into doing things you don't want to do and which you find distasteful, you would become little more than a sex-object used in lust by a number of people and this is not what the sex act is about. It would *not* bring you closer. If he respected you or had any feelings for you he would not want to share you with anyone. He wants you to do something which is the whim of the moment (a degraded whim, I might add), and if you go along with it it won't be long before he treats you like a doormat. So don't be afraid of losing him. There are better men than this, decent men who would appreciate the real you and this is what you deserve. Sex is an act of love between two people who care about each other and your boyfriend definitely does not care about you.'

SEX AFTER MARRIAGE

Teenagers are not the only ones who write to me with problems concerning sex. Even after years of happy marriage, sex can create conflicts, as Madge writes:

'I have been married for five years to a wonderful man
and have three lovely children. My husband and I
communicate well and we are all very happy. The only
hitch that troubles me is our sex life which used to be
very spontaneous and enjoyable for the first few years,
but now seems to be fizzing out. I have taken into
account stress, children and financial problems, but I
feel that my husband is becoming a bit complacent.
When sex is good is always seems to be at my
instigation and imagination. It seems to be a bit
one-sided with me making all the effort and my partner
reaping all the benefits. This leaves me feeling a bit

discontented and cranky. Could you please recommend
some books for my husband and me to read? I want us
to rekindle the spark we once had.'

Madge's feelings are understandable. Many of the sexual problems in marriage come about through mismatched libido. Loss
of libido is a symptom of some sort of breakdown in the way we
relate in other areas, perhaps by both being busy so time isn't
made for one another anymore. Perhaps it is just a part of the
ebb and flow in marriage.

'You are very perceptive and wise to seek help early. If it is
ignored and allowed to continue, this sort of deterioration can
kill a marriage. Your husband may be under pressure of some
kind — perhaps a fear of waning powers with the resulting loss
of self-esteem. Your taking the initiative so often could be
adding to the pressure he feels although in most cases a sexy
wife is a real turn-on.

'I advise you to seek professional help. Get in touch with
ASSERT (Australian Society of Sex Educators, Researchers and
Therapists) [In Sydney, their telephone number is: 665 6660. In
all other states get in touch with Family Planning who would
refer you to a reliable sex counsellor.] An excellent book would
be: *Man, Woman and Sexual Desire*, by Warwick Williams, but
a book alone will not solve your problem. Talking together about
your feelings and needs would be a good therapy to start with.
Loving words often lead to loving encounters.'

Marion's letter illustrates how lack of honesty about one's feelings can create problems that could have been avoided.

'I'm 21 and have been married for three years. I'm very
happy except for one thing — sex. My husband enjoys
it but during intercourse I feel nothing at all and can
hardly wait for it to be over. Last week I worked up
enough courage to tell my husband this, hoping he'd
understand and help me. But instead he was very
angry. So now I don't know what to do. It seems I've
wrecked my marriage by being honest.'

'The shock for your husband probably lay in three years of blissful ignorance that anything was wrong', I replied. 'You generously, but perhaps misguidedly, gave the impression that he was a great lover who always gave you pleasure. A lot of women who are unawakened sexually believe this is the best way of coping with a husband's sexual needs. But it isn't. Sooner or later their own needs demand satisfaction, and when they're expressed, as yours were, you get the angry reaction of the bruised male ego. But at least the way is now open for improvement, whereas while you pretended that everything was fine, there could be no change at all.

'As quickly as you can, correct any impression you may have given that you're accusing him of failing as a lover. Let him see it is a shared problem. Tell him what you would like and if things don't improve, get in touch with Marriage Guidance or your Community Health Centre for counselling help. The present crisis offers a very big challenge to improve sex for both of you.'

Liz wrote:

> 'My husband keeps telling me that my sex drive is very low because I only like intercourse once a week. We've been married for 18 months and it's got to the stage now when he won't come to bed until the early hours of the morning. I love him very much and, if he's right, how can I change my sex drive?'

'Sex drive is something that depends on age and experience, where you are, how you are, and who you're with. So your husband's accusations are his way of saying that, for some reason, you don't seem to want him as much as he wants you. It would be more sensible to look at the reasons for this sad coldness which is building up between you instead of fighting about it. He feels sexually rejected — that's why he's trying to reject you. You have to reassure him that you find him attractive. Why not contact a marriage guidance counsellor?'

Rebecca was feeling guilty about sexual fantasies:

> 'I'm happily married with a three-year-old son. My

problem is that I have sexual fantasies about various
men — some are friends of my husband, others are
strangers. Although my marriage means everything to
me, I'm afraid I'll do something I may regret. Please
give me some wise advice.'

I could tell her that there was absolutely nothing wrong with
her having fantasies. The whole point of fantasies is that they are
a substitute for real sexual behaviour. What every kind of sex life
you find yourself dreaming about — more romantic or more
imaginative — you can create in your love-life.

'Just start using your fantasies with your husband instead of
being frightened of them.'

FEAR OF IMPOTENCE

'We thought that every good thing was coming to us all
at once — new baby, new house, new job that I was
aiming for and really enjoy, and a great marriage. But
now, at the early age of 38, I've become impotent. I'm
desperate about this and so is my wife. Does this mean
the end to our sex life?'

I could reassure him. 'There's no need to panic,' I wrote. 'It's
utterly unjustified and I bet it's based on one, perhaps two
unsuccessful attempts at making love. That is normal in the life
of any man. Potency is a delicate barometer of a man's stresses
and strains. Change of any kind, however welcome and happy is
a stress, and you've had three major ones — new baby, new
house and new job. You have also recently seen your wife go
through childbirth and may feel concerned about hurting her.
Just give yourself a bit of time and everything will be fine.'

Women sometimes write to me about their partner's loss of
libido. Here is such a letter from Lisa:

'Over the past two years my husband has lost interest
in sex. He is 34 and I'm 27 and we only make love two
or three times a month. He went to a doctor because I
insisted, and the doctor said there was nothing wrong

and that a holiday would do him good. We had our
holiday six months ago, and nothing's changed. He says
he knows plenty of guys his age with the same
problem, so it must be because of their age. He won't
see a doctor again. I hope you can help as this whole
problem is getting me down.'

'Now that you have been assured your husband has nothing
physically wrong with him, you would be well-advised to try
another approach to what you see as a problem in your sex-life.
There could be many reasons for your husband's reduced sex-
drive. Desire ebbs and flows and couples don't always have the
same desires or needs at the same time. Men and women get
anxious, moody, tired and depressed now and then, all or any of
which can bring about a fluctuation of desire. Just like anything
else, sex can become boring and then it can become good again.
Personal or business worries, or difficulty in relating to others
can affect one's sexual life — and so can the belief that one is
over the hill and a failure as a lover.

'Perhaps your husband has a weaker sex-drive than you, but if
you continue to make out there is something wrong with him,
you will only reinforce any problem that might exist. A better
approach would be to see what you can do to make your love-life
more enjoyable. Stop thinking about norms — there aren't any
— and focus on love, warmth and fun.'

MOTHERHOOD AND SEX

Over the years I have read many letters like this one from Debra.

'I'm 21, happily married and have an adorable son of
two months. During my pregnancy, intercourse meant
nothing to me so we stopped, thinking that after the
baby was born everything would be fine. But I'm just
the same and I'm afraid my husband will become tired
of waiting and find another woman. He never says
anything about it but I know it's upsetting him and it
makes me upset too.'

It is only natural that an event such as motherhood with all its physical, emotional, and hormonal changes must make a difference to a woman's feelings about sex — not necessarily better or worse, but different.

'Are you both expecting your sex life to be the same as before — that or nothing? Relax and be sensitive to the change in you both. Keeping silent about it is the worse thing you can do. Talk about it honestly and frankly and before long you'll find that you are becoming closer and your loving will lead to making love.'

Tony wrote about a problem which is much more common than is imagined.

> 'We're expecting our first child in two months and I want the baby as much as my wife does. But our sex-life has stopped and, I'm ashamed to say, the reason is that I can't bear her near me in bed since the baby started moving. I find the kicks rather "spooky" and very off-putting. I've tried to explain, but she thinks I no longer love her.'

'There's no need to feel ashamed — this is not an uncommon reaction in a father-to-be,' I wrote back. 'But this is a time when your wife does need extra reassurance that she's not unattractive. And she certainly needs to be sure of your love. A peaceful mind is most important to her well-being and also to the baby's. I might add that the way you relate to her now will have a far-reaching effect on your relationship. A feeling of rejection or of being let down at this time, seems to hurt women very deeply. So couldn't you demonstrate your love, even if sex is out of the question? There are many ways of embracing and touching. Just as important, there are many loving and caring words too.'

HOMOSEXUALITY

Homosexuality, once a taboo subject, is now 'out of the closet', but there is still a lot of ignorance and misinformation on the part of heterosexuals as to what being 'gay' actually means.

I receive many letters from people who are afraid they may be gay because of feelings and impulses they experience and don't understand. Each of us, whether male or female, has both a male and a female side to our personalities. One side is nurturing and sensitive; the other, ambitious and more confident. Some people show both sides of their personalities; others let one side dominate. Ideally, the most balanced men and women are those who allow both sides of their personalities to show. Women are now acknowledging their practical side in business, and men are allowing their sensitive, nurturing side to come through.

Often people who doubt their own sexuality, mistrust their feelings and think they must be 'different'. Another aspect of this is the need we all have for love and nurturing through our lives and more so when we are babies. If we are deprived of this love, or don't get as much or it as we like, we end up with a deficit need which drives us to search for it in every relationship. We can get the grown-up version in the form of caring and acknowledgment from a parent, a lover, a spouse or friend. Many people who write to me sometimes mistake this normal, human need to be loved in a non-sexual way as a sign that they are gay.

Another group who write to me are those who fear they may be gay on the strength of one experience. They need to give themselves some time and experience relationships with both sexes if possible, before they can define their sexuality.

There is still a lot we do not know about homosexuality, but we do know that in the past homosexuals have been unjustly blamed for many wrongs. For instance, child molesters are not homosexuals as a rule, nor are most transvestites.

My area of help is to point out the wealth of information available now: reading matter, specialised counselling and consultation, and the support groups which did not exist a few years ago. Anyone in need of counselling can get in touch with ASSERT (Australian Society of Sex Educators, Researchers and Therapists), tel: (02) 665 6660. In other states it is best to contact your Family Planning Association or a similar body and they will refer you to a reliable sex therapist.

The first letter is from Brad:

'I am a 20-year-old man, and I think I'm gay. I often find myself fantasising about males, more than I do females. I don't want to be gay, I just want to be a

normal heterosexual guy. I would definitely never
involve myself in a homosexual relationship, but I need
to kill these fantasies so that I can have peace of mind.
When I do have sex with a girl, I really enjoy it, but it
only lasts while we are together physically. Please help
me, Kate.'

'The more you resist your fantasies, the more they will persist, as you are finding out', I wrote. 'It is a fact that many heterosexual males have homosexual fantasies, so perhaps you are being too hard on yourself. It is not unnatural at your age to have fantasies such as these in your struggle to find a sexual identity. You seem to be fighting something you think is horrific, and this is why you can't get rid of your recurring thoughts.

'If you could be more accepting of yourself, whatever your sexual preferences, you might find the problem taking on a more balanced perspective. While in our society it is more acceptable to be heterosexual, you would not suddenly become a monster if you discovered you were homosexual. Why not try behaviour therapy which has been used in cases such as yours? Ask about it in a large hospital near you. But the very first step which you can take this minute is to accept yourself as a unique and valuable human being no matter what.'

Samantha wrote:

'I'm 16 and I don't like boys because I'm a lesbian. I
keep way from the girls I like at school so they won't
find out about my real feelings. But there's a married
woman with a little boy who lives near me. I love her
and visit her every day after school. Could she feel the
same about me? Can a married woman with a child
have lesbian feelings?'

'I beg you to stop putting your loving feelings into these narrow little pigeonholes,' I replied, 'as if sexual love was the only kind there is. Your dislike of boys, affection for your friends and love for this woman (plus a variety of other feelings for other people) are part of the wide range of constantly changing emotions explored by every growing person.

'The deep affection you feel for this woman is probably a yearning you have to be loved and mothered in the same way you see her mothering her three-year-old. If subconsciously you feel you missed out on that kind of nurturing, it is only natural to look for it no matter what your age. You don't have to look at every relationship as a potentially sexual one. By giving you her time and acknowledgment, this lady is giving you the grown-up version of that love we need in infancy.

'And you are missing out on what could be good friendships with the girls at school if you would simply accept that it is normal to feel strongly for your own sex sometimes — for their companionship, their closeness, their support. So just relax and give your feelings time to grow and settle.'

Fiona wrote:

'I'm 19. For the past three years it's been girls and
women I've dreamed about and fallen for, not men,
although it's always been at a distance. Now there's a
girl at work, who is the same age as me. I really like
her. But I try to avoid her in case she's not "different"
like me. I am so lonely it's driving me round the twist.
As I'll never be able to have a boyfriend, how can I
make a few friends so that I can go out and enjoy
myself like them?'

'If this is your first attempt at a real relationship, as distinct from crushes on strangers, you just can't know where you really stand in the heterosexual/homosexual spectrum until you've made contact with people of both sexes and found out whether it is timidity about males or a real preference for your own sex, that's creating all your confusion. An attempt to make friends with this girl can't do any harm. You could find that neither of you wants to turn it into a love-affair. She could even help you solve some of your problems — social life is much easier in pairs and with her back-up it would be easier to make other friendships. If you really are homosexual it will become apparent through experience and not through just thinking about yourself and wondering.'

INCEST — THE NEW TABOO

Claire's problem was one which I first mentioned in my 'closed file' in the seventies, but now is gradually being spoken about.

> 'I am 20 years of age and live with my fiancé. When I
> was very young I was a victim of incest. I often wake
> up during the night and start hitting into my fiancé
> thinking he is either my brother or my father who is
> dead now. Sometimes my fiancé has to hold me down to
> calm me. He wants to know what is wrong and is very
> understanding, but I don't know how to tell him, and
> if I did tell him, how he would feel about me?'

I knew Claire needed counselling from someone who was specialised in this particular area but I wanted her to know she had my understanding.

'There must be a great deal of anger and hurt in you which needs to be expressed — but not to someone very close to you, not yet, anyway. You need to talk to a professional counsellor specialising in your particular kind of problem. I urge you to ring either or both of the following help agencies. There is the Child Abuse Prevention Society in NSW (it is not only for children who are being abused, but also children who were abused years ago.) Another organisation in NSW is Dympna House — tel: (02) 797 6733.

You've taken the first step in writing to me — and that would have given you a measure of relief. Now take it a step further and seek professional help.'

Lisa's letter was an unhappy example of what happens so often in cases of sexual abuse within the family.

> 'I'm 16 and am worried by the way my 23-year-old
> brother plays around with me when we're alone —
> which is far from brotherly. He has no girlfriends. I
> can't do anything to stop him as he's very strong. I
> don't lead him on in any way. Why does he behave like
> this?'

Sexual interest between brothers and sisters is not unusual in childhood, when it is largely prompted by curiosity. But we usually grow out of this and a natural barrier arises. Your brother clearly hasn't grown out of it, even though you are both at an age to develop relationships and activiteis outside the family. You must obviously avoid being in the house alone with him too often and for too long. And you must tell your parents, so they can get some help for your brother.

Emma's letter was only one of many I receive on this same theme. She wrote:

'I'm 15 and desperate. My father makes me have sex with him when my mother is at work. If I don't he bashes me and threatens to put me in a home. Can you help me? I don't know which way to turn?'

I wished Emma had given me an address. All I could do was answer through my column.

'Take no notice of your father's threats,' I wrote. 'If the police were informed of his abuse he would be prosecuted by law. Can you go to the police in your area? If you can't, I urge you to go to your family doctor, or to a minister of religion or a priest and tell them what you have written to me. They would take the necessary steps to protect you from this man's assaults. In the meantime, can you be out of the house when he is at home? Do you have a relative, or even a friend you can stay with? But for heaven's sake don't just stand there and take this shocking abuse.'

Rebecca's letter was one of the saddest I have read.

'I can't keep going through life the way I am. I can't hold a job for more than a few months. I make mistakes, forget things, argue with the boss and keep thinking the people I work with are talking about me. I go off in a day-dream and can't snap out of it. When I have a boyfriend, after a few weeks I get jealous and take over their lives, we argue all the time and they leave. I can't keep friends and I can't even stabilise my weight. I also have a history of trying to kill myself. I

have been sexually abused and bashed — first by my
father, then by my stepfather — and it has been going
on for as long as I remember until three years ago. I
get so depressed, feel evil, and my mind is tormented.
Where can I go for help? Is there any hope?

'Of course there is hope for you,' I wrote back. 'You have such
a clear insight into your problems I am confident you will overcome them and make a good life for yourself. The sexual abuse
will have left deep emotional scars. Now you need to see a
counsellor — preferably a woman — who is experienced in
these matters and who will give you all the understanding you
need to get it out of your system and find peace of mind. All the
other problems you have in relating, whether at work, with a
boyfriend or with friends, stem from your basic insecurities.
Everything in your life will improve when you get to the heart of
what is destroying you. Get in touch with any large hospital near
you and ask for the Sexual Assault Centre (or Rape Centre).
You've taken the first big step in writing to me. Now follow
through and take the steps which will make life good again.'

This last letter from Jacki shows one of the more devious ways in
which sexual assault can manifest itself.

'I am 14 years old and I want to leave home because of
my father. Every time I play up, give cheek or do
something wrong, my father puts me across his knee
and spanks me. Sometimes he even smacks my bare
bottom which I find very humiliating as well as
painful. I have complained to my mother a few times
but she just says I get what I deserve and that if I
didn't misbehave, I wouldn't get spanked. While I admit
I'm no angel, I just wish I could get grounded or sent
to my room like the other kids at school. Can you
please help me, Kate?'

'I would not advise you to leave home just yet — it would not
be in your best interests,' I wrote back. 'But you need to confide
in someone about what is happening. Do you have a school

counsellor? Or you could get in touch with your nearest Community Health Centre and talk to a counsellor who would understand how you feel. You could also ring the Department of Family and Community Services. What your father is doing constitutes assault with sexual overtones and should be stopped at once. Don't feel guilty about getting outside help. You tried your mother and your plea was ignored. Now *you* must do something to stop this humiliating abuse.'

This letter from Brett touched me deeply.

'I have spent much of the past 20 years in turmoil over an episode that occurred in my youth. Relatives came to live near us when I was 17. Soon my cousin, who had just turned 11, was spending most of her time at our place and what started as playful rolling in the grass, eventually led to intercourse.

This went on for some months until my uncle's work meant moving overseas. I have not seen her since, but kept track through family gossip.

I recently found out that she lost her husband in an accident and will be returning to Australia with her two children and will be living quite near to my home. I knew from the start that what I was doing was wrong and spent years in fear of being found out. As adulthood and maturity came, these fears subsided and I became worried about the effect this episode may have had on her life.

Over the past six years this has become an obsession, with bouts of depresson and thoughts of suicide. I have been successful in my work and two years ago I started a trust fund for her children and made her sole beneficiary of my estate. (I have no living direct relatives.) We have never been in contact, although she has occasionally asked about me in letters to an aunt. I don't know what to do. Should I stay away or offer help? I do not want to upset her further.'

I felt he had suffered enough for his mistake and needed support and reassurance.

'You appear very distressed and conscious-stricken about events which happened so long ago. It is right for you to feel responsible for your part in what took place. Meeting her now might help you both. However, I suggest that you seek counselling for your depression and distress over past mistakes. Get in touch with your nearest community health centre and ask to see someone who is experienced in these matters. After speaking to them you may have a clearer idea about what you'd like to say to your cousin.'

9

When In-laws are Outlaws

ADAM, SO WE ARE TOLD, was the luckiest man in creation because he was the only one without in-laws. Leaving such jokes aside, it is a fact that each partner has two families — spouse and children make up one family, parents and brothers and sisters make up the other. Maintaining a harmonious balance between the two is a difficult task.

For a well-adjusted person, their own spouse and children will come first and their family of origin second. Unfortunately, some men and women never quite make the emotional break with their parents and many parents never really let go of their children, and this is where problems arise. On the other hand, complete exclusion of one's parents and siblings is also a sign of immaturity and unresolved conflicts. As with any other relationship, the in-law connection requires compromise and diplomacy, plus a lot of goodwill.

Until a few years ago, most of the letters I received dealing with in-law troubles were about the conflict between a daughter-in-law and her husband's mother. Often it was the mother who was jealous and rejected the younger woman for taking away her son. Just as often the younger woman was jealous of the natural bond between mother and son and was threatened by it. As always in such situations, the meat in the sandwich was the man concerned, trying to be a loyal husband and loving son.

My aim is to get both women to see the other's point of view. To the mother I'd say:

'You are older and wiser and have more understanding of what life is about. Remember back to the time you were a young bride and how you felt when criticised by your husband's mother. Treat your son's wife as you wish you had been treated.' To the younger woman I always said: 'You and your husband have your young lives ahead of you, a future of love and dreams to realise together. Your mother-in-law feels she has lost the man who was once her little boy. No matter how happy she is to see her son happy with you, she knows her life is behind her and that brings a sense of loss which can come across as rejection. You can afford to be generous and let her see that although you must make your own lives, she is still much-loved and respected. Make her your friend, not your enemy. After all, you both love the same man.'

I always tried to show that love is not about possession. It grows in an atmosphere of mutual sharing and acceptance.

FAMILY FEUDS

Alison wrote:

'I am 22 and engaged to a very caring 28-year-old guy. The problem is both our parents. They simply don't get on and seem to dislike one another and shared visits always end in argument. My fiancé and I are both very upset and distressed by their attitude and behaviour and we are at a loss as to what we can do about it. Our relationship is being affected and if it continues after we are married I know it will cause rows between us. We love each other very much but all this is making us unhappy and tense. What can we do?'

'Of course you'd be happier if they got on well', I said, 'but what you need to realise is that your relationship with your fiancé is the important one and not the relationship between the in-laws, however much you'd like that to be good. It will help you to understand that when parents are losing their children to marriage, they go through many insecurities and misconceptions. You and your fiancé could reassure both sets of parents that because you are marrying you haven't changed sides, that they are still loved and respected as much as ever. But be firm in pointing out that you must make your own lives regardless of their unwillingness to let you go. Both of you have a private chat with your respective parents and tell them it's OK to have differences and not to get on, but it's not OK to have fights. Ask them to agree to a little social politeness and don't invite them to get together. If you and your fiancé can have a laugh at their childish behaviour and not be affected by it, you'll find that it will settle down eventually.'

Sara's letter told of an unusual situation.

'I have always been on good terms with my husband's parents, especially my mother-in-law whom I regard as a good friend. Now my husband has fallen out with them over a business deal and is not on speaking terms with them. He has every reason to be angry, but his mother swears there was no ill-intent, that things just turned out badly, that's all. But my husband says I must not speak to his family and that I must stay away from them. We have three children whom the grandparents love dearly. How can I deprive them of this pleasure? Yet I don't want to go behind my husband's back, although I disagree with his ideas. Surely, adults don't have to behave in this way?'

Ideally, adults should be forgiving and mature, but we are all human and so we react according to the way we feel. However, Sara must make her husband understand that although she is on his side, she disagrees with his attitude towards his parents and refuses to involve the children in his petty vendetta. Sara can get her message across and still show him she cares about him.
'I am sure his anger will soon pass and he will be just as glad as you to be friends with his family.'

Maggie's problem is one I hear often:

'My husband doesn't like my parents and I'm gradually being torn in two by efforts to keep the peace. I'm an only child and my parents live half an hour's drive

away. They like to come and see me and our three
children when they feel like it, sometimes in the late
afternoon during the week, and sometimes during the
weekend. My husband says they must only come when
they are invited but he never wants to invite them.
The atmosphere is really terrible if he's already here or
comes home during their visits. What should I do?'

'Would it make your husband happier if you showed your real
willingness to compromise a little and if the visits were fewer
and better-timed?

'You see, it may not be the actual visits which annoy him, but
the fact that you are still too emotionally tied to them in a
childish way. No man likes to feel he comes second in this kind
of situation, so your gesture would leave it open for your husband, too, to compromise. Then you could both decide together
when they could visit. His idea of inviting them could be the
answer, for it is the only way of having the frequency of the visits
under both your and his control instead of under the sole control
of your parents. This is a natural wish for most families at home,
no matter how deep the affection they have for relatives.'

LIVING WITH IN-LAWS

Nancy's letter is one of many on the topic of living with parents
for a time while saving for their own home.

'I am getting married next year to a wonderful guy
whom I love very much. We have bought a block of
land and hope to build a house on it, but would like to
save a bit more money. My fiancé wants us to live with
his parents for a year after we are married. My sister
did the same thing and she couldn't stand living with
her in-laws. When I told my fiancé about her
experience, he just said that his parents are different.
Would this kind of arrangement work out?'

I replied that in general I don't think young marrieds should
live with their in-laws, but that Nancy's fiancé was right — her
experience will not necessarily be the same as her sister's.

'I am also assuming that you will be going out to work, which will make it easier. The domestic situation you are considering will work well if you discuss it beforehand with them, especially your fiancé's mother, and come to an agreement as to the house rules. You need to agree that everything will be up front. If you get on each other's nerves, you will need to discuss it and not let it smoulder in silent resentment. How much privacy and how much togetherness should be decided, and what is expected in the way of chores and pitching in. I suggest you occasionally make thoughtful gestures to your mother-in-law, for instance, a bunch of flowers or whatever you know she likes. If you and your husband are sensitive to each other's needs as well as to his parents' needs, I think the arrangement can work for a year.

THE INTERFERING MOTHER-IN-LAW

The problem expressed in Nikki's letter is a common one:

'We have been married for ten months, are very much in love and everything would be perfect if it were not for one thing: my mother-in-law seems to think no one can look after her son (my husband) as well as she did. She makes snide remarks and comments which make me seem hopeless at everything. He is her only child and she's a widow so I suppose she is finding it hard to let go, but her interference is causing us to quarrel a lot. I love my husband and don't want to hurt him but do I have to become a doormat to his mother?'

'This is a tricky situation but by no means a hopeless one,' I replied. 'You don't have to become a doormat, but you have a very important lesson to learn and it's this: how to make your mother-in-law your friend instead of your enemy. And how do you do this? You listen to what she says without reacting, you admit you don't know all there is to know (even if you think you do), and ask for help and advice to put it right. She'll be flattered and amazed at how perceptive you are, and will immediately be on side with you. But you don't have to take the advice. All you have to do is listen and appear to be grateful. Later on when you feel more secure in yourself and your marriage, you may find that some of the advice is worth taking. By doing this you will not be a hypocrite, just diplomatic!'

Beth wrote:

> 'I have a wonderful husband and a lovely baby girl. But my mother-in-law is spoiling everything. She's always phoning my husband for help — and when she does, he drops everything and goes to her house. She keeps telling us how we should run our lives and it seems nothing I do is right in her eyes. Her own husband is completely downtrodden and never utters a word. When she and I have an argument my husband takes sides with her at the time but usually agrees with me afterwards. I'm really beginning to feel second-best and it's making me unhappy. I often feel like leaving my husband, but I love him so much and I know he loves me and our baby.'

'Your mother-in-law sounds very demanding,' I replied, 'but I'm sure you are reacting more to her interference now because of the arrival of your baby. It's only natural that you want your husband more in the home now, so his rushing off to his mother's house makes you feel more neglected and, as you put it, "second-best". And of course, I can understand how sensitive you must be as a young mother to unsolicited advice which undermines your self-confidence in being able to cope.

'I'm afraid your mother-in-law isn't about to change her ways, so, what you must not do is let it become an issue between you and your husband. I am sure he loves you both, though in different ways, of course. In his mother's case his love may be mixed with a lot of fear, because of her bossiness and desire to control everyone.

'Instead of battling with her, concentrate on maintaining a loving warmth and harmony between you and your husband — particularly in front of her, even if it means appearing to accept her point of view when you actually don't. Making no comment is sometimes the loudest comment of all. You can listen to someone's advice, after all, without having to act on it. She simply can't rule your lives if you and your husband have a calm, united certainty about what you want to do, and the way you want to do it.

'Above all don't place your husband in a position where he must choose between you and his mother in an argument. Sometimes you win by appearing to lose.'

By far the most common problem between daughters-in-law and their husband's mother has to do with unwanted advice from the older woman. Here is Emma's letter.

'Until I came home with my new baby son, I got on well with my mother-in-law. She likes me a lot and I like her so there was never any trouble. But now she's at our place very day giving me non-stop advice on how to bring up our son. Her ideas are very old-fashioned, of course, and I find myself disagreeing with her all the time. I don't want repeated arguments as they upset me. Shall I tell her I'd like to do things my way?'

'Don't you think that would sound harsh and hurtful to someone who appears to be basically kind?' I asked. 'Try to accept the advice in the spirit in which it is offered, keeping in mind that you don't have to do as she suggests if you don't agree with it. As for your methods or hers, they are neither right nor wrong, just different. After all, she reared your husband by her methods and he's perfectly all right, isn't he? Did you know that some of the older methods of child-rearing, relying on a mother's instinct, are now being re-considered as the ideal? The strictly clinical approach taught in recent years has been found to be more harmful than the older method. So why not discuss and compare these different ways instead of arguing and being resentful? A bit of humour always helps. And you may find as time goes by that having her as an ally and a back-up will benefit you and your son — and your husband too.'

LIVE-IN MOTHERS-IN-LAW

Marion writes about a problem which is affecting more and more people today.

'Now that my husband's mother is a widow, she feels
she should come to live with us. My husband is an
only child and she has lived her life only for him, so
she hasn't any friends or interests. We get on OK, but
frankly, I couldn't cope with her living with us as she
is a very domineering person. The children don't want
her to come. My mother is alone too, and she copes
very well, but she'd be hurt if I agreed to have my
mother-in-law to live with us. How can I best handle
this without hurting anyone?'

This is a difficult situation and Marion won't solve it without a
few bruised feelings.

'Unless your mother-in-law is old and frail or in poor health,' I
wrote, 'there is no reason why she should live with you. She is
probably no more than middle-aged, in which case she is not
too old to make new friends and develop new interests. If there
were an outlet for her energy, she might not be so domineering
and obsessed with her son. Try to let her see the disadvantages
(for her) of living in a home with children — the noise, the
constant activity and demands, and the lack of privacy. Perhaps if
you invited her to stay for a week during the school holidays, she
might decide that living alone has many compensations! In any
case, try not to become her enemy. It would help if you got her
interested in some activity where she would enjoy the company
of people of her own generation. Try not to let yourself be
stampeded into making a decision against your inclination and
judgement. You can be firm, yet still be kind.'

Jerry wrote:

'My wife's mother has just been widowed. Although
she's an active, independent woman, the only answer to
her accommodation problem is that she comes to live
with us. We have enough room, but I dread her
intrusion into the very happy, full lives my wife and I
lead now that I'm retired. We travel around a lot by
caravan and I'd be really miserable if we had to stop
doing this.'

'Why should your trips have to stop?' I wanted to know. 'There may have to be a little more forethought and planning, perhaps more keeping in touch by phone while you're away, but no more change than that. She wouldn't want your lives intermingled with hers any more than you would — her independence is just as important to her. It is necessary that you get the practical basis of your living together very clearly marked out from the start — who pays for what, eating arrangements, what is separate and what is shared territory. That makes for more amicable living.'

June's letter shows what can happen when a strong mother-in-law is allowed to dominate.

> 'My marriage has been very happy until a month ago when my husband's mother came to live with us. She's taken over the house and does the cooking, always preparing the dishes she prefers or what she thinks we ought to eat. She and my husband go out in her car while I'm working and they don't talk to me much when we're home. I feel really pushed out. I can't tell her to go as it would cause trouble, and besides, I don't actually dislike her.'

I felt that June's problem was with her husband and not his mother, and I tried to find a way of telling her so tactfully.

'No matter how dominating a woman may be, she can't take over a married son and his home, as she's doing, unless he allows her to. So you need to work out with your husband a plan of some sort that's not going to make any of you feel unwanted or miserable. It won't be easy! It's a situation he'll have to make clear to his mother if she's to stay living with you and it will take a lot of understanding and goodwill and tact. But you might also try looking on the positive side. Many women who go out to work would love to come home to a cooked meal. Just make sure she cooks what you and your husband like most of the time. Encourage her to make friends of her own age group and to have a few interests outside the home. This would channel some of her energy into constructive activity and make her less domineering. Let her know she is free to invite friends to lunch or a cup of tea and a chat any time she wants.

'And you must make time to be with your husband so that you don't feel pushed out. If you can relax and stop resisting having your mother-in-law in the house, your relationship with him and her will improve more than you imagine.'

THE IMPORTANCE OF BEING HONEST

Jenny wrote:

'Although we both love having my husband's mother to stay with us every month, we're both helpless at letting her know what suits us, so she always ends up outstaying her welcome. Once she stayed a fortnight when four days would have suited us, and her too, I suspect. She's a widow so I don't want to hurt her feelings, but what can *I do?*'

'You're so nice — but so vague that you end up hurting her as well as yourself,' I wrote. 'It's much better to have a definite arrangement from the start. I bet she'd rather know the limit of her stay than hang on past her welcome. So next time you ask her say, "We'd like you to come on Friday and stay until Tuesday if you can."'

The question of hospitality is one which many older parents find difficult to handle. This letter from Gwen says it all:

'My husband retired last year and we live in the home we've lived in for 35 years. It's all paid for, has a lovely garden and we manage all right financially, as long as it's just us. But we have five children and 12 grandchildren who visit us often, sometimes bringing friends too. I hate to admit it but it's getting beyond us to provide food, drink and everything that goes with good hospitality. We often go short between our 'entertaining' in order to do things properly. They always bring flowers — but we grow enough to give away, and anyway, you can't serve flowers as a first course, can you? We've gone over this problem endlessly and have come to the reluctant conclusion that the

only answer is to ask the family to come less often.
But it breaks our hearts to think of it as we love them
all so much and they love coming, so is there any
solution, Kate?'

'Yes there is,' I answered, 'and it's to be absolutely honest with
your family. How can they know their visits cripple you if you
entertain them lavishly, sparing nothing? Perhaps you think they
should guess the truth, knowing you're pensioners, but most of
us take things at face value, and if you give the appearance of
being flush by giving what you consider "proper" hospitality, it
does not even occur to them to look deeper. When they know
how things really are with you, I'm sure they'll be glad to bring
food and drink with them instead of flowers, and you can all
continue to enjoy these visits.'

BLUDGING RELATIVES

This next problem has cropped up intermittently over the years,
sometimes with variations where it's the country relatives who
feel put upon! Shirley wrote:

'Why do country relatives think their city family are at
their beck and call to provide board and lodging
whenever they want it?

'My husband and I are tired of having these bludgers
taking over every long weekend and annual holiday,
loud and clear on the subject of food preferences, using
the phone at every whim, watching their favourite TV
programs and, in general, being obnoxious. They do not
lift a finger to help in any way or provide anything.

The cost to us financially and emotionally is
astronomical. Wake up visitors! Why do you think we
never stay with you?'

In my reply I pointed out the part Shirley and her husband
had played in the situation.

'The fear of hurting other people's feelings without ever considering your own always ends up working against you, as you
are finding out. It does not do *them* any good, either. Inconsid-
erate people become that way because no one ever tells them

that what they are doing is unacceptable. They will only begin to learn when someone calls a halt and says "no".

'I am not advocating that we always put ourselves first and ignore others, only that we treat ourselves with the same respect as anyone else. You don't have to be nasty to your relatives. A simple "we have made other plans and it would not be convenient for you to come and stay at this time" is a statement which is not offensive. It will be difficult the first few times, since you have not had any practice at it, but it does get easier.

'Your family will have to cope with their feelings. It's clear to me that it is this fear of hurting them which probably goes back a long time, which has made you so unassertive. You can change, you know, and when you do, you'll find that you will enjoy their occasional visits at your convenience.'

MISUNDERSTOOD MOTHERS-IN-LAW

Although it is mostly daughters-in-law who write to me, there is a fair sprinkling of letters from mothers-in-law.

Tess's letter is an example of what happens when we assume we know what the other person is thinking.

> 'I've never been able to put my finger on what is actually wrong, but my daughter-in-law and I are completely out of tune with each other. I never seem to do the right thing when I visit her home, so I only go three or four times a year, just so that I don't lose touch with my son. But it upsets and depresses me very much not to see more of my family. They have three children whom I love dearly, and I miss not being able to enjoy their company more, but I don't want to be accused of butting in, so there's nothing I can do.'

'But there is, you know,' I replied. 'You may not want to visit more often, but what is there to stop you from inviting your grandchildren to stay with you occasionally during their holidays? You could go on special outings with them and enjoy their company. You could also invite your son and daughter-in-law to visit you.

'It sounds as if there is some misunderstanding between you which will not be cleared up by silence on both sides. You are older and wiser, so ask your daughter-in-law to sit quietly with you at some stage and talk with her (not *at* her). Say: "Look, I feel there are barriers between us which prevent us from being close and it makes me sad. Would you like to tell me why you need to hold back? What don't you like about me?" Then listen and be willing to hear the answer. When she's finished you can say: "I'll tell you how I feel about you". You will need a lot of tact and what you say must be in the cause of better understanding and not an opportunity to tell each other off. You will find many truths if you use such honesty although it may not all happen in one go. But you must create the opening for anything to change. It's no good going on for years with the tacit agreement: "We don't get on". Before you talk, pick out an incident or an instance and ask yourself: "What did I do, what did I contribute to this situation, what did *we* do?", then talk to her about it. You can heal the rift if you are both willing. Just lead the way.'

IN-LAWS KEEP THEIR DISTANCE

In this next letter from Liz, we see how difficult it is to strike a happy balance between too much and too little attention from a mother-in-law.

'I live 100 yards from my in-laws and always felt they were good friends. Four months ago I had my first baby and he was very colicky. I found this very exhausting and frustrating. The night after I came home from hospital they came to visit and have only popped in about twice since for no more than five minutes. I really needed their help and moral support as I have no family nearby and would have appreciated them coming to watch my baby or play with him for an hour or so so that I could catch up with some housework and get some shopping done. I was hurt as they always make such a big deal over him and buy expensive gifts for him. I feel very bitter over their lack of concern for my son and myself. I hate feeling this way and don't know what to do as I don't want to rock the boat since we live so close.

> 'They have two other grandchildren (girls) and were
> most excited about a grandson. My sister-in-law and her
> family also live next door and her feelings are similar
> to mine. I am not overly close to my sister-in-law and
> family, but there is no hostility. I am 22-years-old and
> the baby is now over his colic.'

I answered: 'Perhaps your in-laws are lacking in awareness
and thoughtfulness, but I feel they are trying so desperately to
be "cool" and not interfere in your life, that they come across as
uncaring. Most of the letters I get from young mums like you
have the opposite problem — they feel their in-laws are trying to
take over their baby and their lives. I'm sure if they knew how
you feel they'd behave differently, so why not ask for the help
you need? It would probably bring you closer. So do it. A word of
advice: don't go discussing them to anyone, especially anyone in
the family, for example, your sister-in-law. If they thought you
were criticising them behind their back it would be the surest
way to rock the boat and lose their trust. Ask for what you want
in a pleasant, direct way and I'm sure you'll get on well.'

VISITING THE IN-LAWS

Christmas is a very special time of the year to be spent with
family and friends — but the obligations we all feel can sometimes be a problem.

> 'I have been married 12 years, have three children, and
> my husband and I are fairly happy except for one bone
> of contention — his mother. Every Christmas he
> expects me to travel thousands of kilometres in the
> heat so that we can have Christmas with his family. We
> stay about a month. His mother is very nasty to me
> and I find it hard to stick the month out — I stand
> her for so long and then flare up and say I'm going
> back home. He always manages to make me stay. But I
> haven't had a holiday for eight years and I think it's
> very unfair of him to expect me to go there every year.
> Should I stick up for myself or become resigned to the
> situation and grin and bear it?'

'You seem to be standing up for yourself, but in the wrong way and at the wrong time', I replied. 'This merely cancels out your efforts which are never heard. This is a subject that should be discussed with your husband when you are both calm and receptive. That is when you are more likely to put your point across rather than in the heat of anger. No doubt you'd like a change in your holiday plans, but could it be that your resentful attitude contributes to your miserable time and your uneasy relationship with your husband's mother?

'Have you considered making other arrangements for the coming year? For instance, you could spend Christmas and a few days with your husband's family and then have a holiday yourself away from them with a friend, perhaps, or whatever you choose. There are many possibilities once you begin to look for them. The secret is to be happy and gracious for the short time you spend with your mother-in-law and then go off and do what you really want to do with a light heart. And yes, it would help if you grinned a little more!'

Becky wrote:

'Whenever we visit my in-laws with our two-year-old son, it's such a strain I come away worn out. We are always made to sit in the kitchen, and all the time my mother-in-law hovers around us with a damp cloth and dustpan and brush at the ready. I've said nothing to my husband about it because I don't want to cause trouble, and apart from all this I know they love me and our son.'

All I could say was that's the way Becky's mother-in-law is and nothing is going to change her.

'But I am sure you could put up with it more easily if you did share it with your husband — not in a complaining way, but just as an interesting insight into his parents' lives and possibly his own childhood. There's also a funny side to it that would secretly lighten the visits for you if you'd let it. Or maybe you could offer to clean up. Just sitting there passively can be harder than doing something to take your mind off it.'

THINK BEFORE YOU SPEAK

Hilda's letter showed clearly how even a few thoughtless words can damage a relationship beyond forgiveness. She wrote:

'I've just had an argument with my son and his wife. My son went overseas for six months and while he was away, I looked after his wife. She used to come over for dinner and visits and so on. I don't like the fact that she didn't thank me for looking after her. On the night of the argument, my son told us that his wife had just had a miscarriage. When he was outside, I said 'I hope she has ten more.' I didn't think he heard me but he told me he did. Now I've alienated the whole family from them. What should I do? My son's wife doesn't forgive easily and after this I fear I may have lost them both forever.'

I tended to agree. 'Yes, your thoughtless, vindictive remark may well have cut too deeply ever to be forgiven, and created more mischief in your family than you intended. You need to look at why you made such a venomous remark at a time when both young people were in a vulnerable state after her miscarriage. Was it because she didn't thank you enough for having her to dinner a few times? Do you really consider this "looking after her"? She is an adult woman and did not need looking after by you or anyone else. And surely, having a family member to dinner is a mutual pleasure and not the big deal you seem to think it is. You do not come across as a generous or loving woman and mother.

'All I can suggest is that you apologise from the bottom of your heart and ask their forgiveness. But only do this if you are genuinely sorry for what you did and not just to smooth things over. Have you learned any lesson from all of this? Unkindness always boomerangs back on the one who is unkind. Eat as much humble pie as you need to eat to let them see you are sorry, and do try to be kinder in the future. I can only hope your son and daughter-in-law are more generous than you are.'

10
Assimilating Can Be Difficult

MY MAIL HAS ALWAYS included a fair percentage of letters from people who have recently settled in Australia. This is not surprising since one in three Australians are born in another country or have parents who came to Australia from another country.

In the early years of my column, the letters were mostly from Italians and Greeks. These days I receive them from many nationalities: Lebanese, Maltese, Thai, Indonesian, Chinese and Japanese. Whatever the nationality, the problems they write to me about come from their difficulty in adjusting to a completely different way of life.

When a person decides to emigrate, they take a quantum leap into the unknown. If the reality they find here is not too different from their expectations, they adjust more easily. But no matter how stable and well-adjusted, few migrants settle without trauma. Often, however, they attribute problems to their migrant status when they are the very same problems faced by any of us — problems with communication, relationships and self-esteem. Of course, if you are a stranger in a strange land, any existing personal problem can become more overwhelming.

When I first began writing for magazines, I received many letters from Italian and Greek women, always complaining of the many restrictions in their lives. They were not allowed to go out alone and even girlfriends were forbidden for fear of them providing a bad example. Occasional letters on this theme still trickle in. When people leave all that is familiar and secure, and are transplanted into a totally different environment and society, they tend to cling together to those who share a similar back-ground and to the old traditions, for support and strength.

Moving to another country creates its own special problems, but there are basic human conflicts which are common to us all, regardless of colour or race. The symptoms may appear to be different, but the causes are the same. All relationships are open to difficulty, but if you choose to enter into a relationship with a person of a different culture you must expect that you may encounter difficulties, springing from your differences. Inevitably, the basic cultural mores you each have are bound to clash. In some cases you can never eradicate these convictions which make compromise practically impossible. But relationships between different races can work if both parties are responsible and face up to the enormous differences involved.

I FEEL LIKE A PRISONER

The first letter, from Maria, arrived only a few months ago. I used to receive many more like it in the early years of my column, but am happy to say I don't get many like it today.

> 'I am 26 years of age and live at home with my
> parents. I am Italian and still single as my father has
> never allowed me to have friends or to go out by
> myself. I have worked in the family business ever since
> I left school. I would like to get married to a nice man
> and start a family of my own but it doesn't look as if
> this will ever happen as I don't meet any Italian men
> where I work. I get very depressed and worry that I
> will become an old maid. Please help me as I think a
> lot about suicide lately.'

'Your desires and wishes for the future are perfectly normal,' I replied. 'It's your parents' attitude which is abnormal in this day and age — and country. They are fearfully looking at life as if they were still living in a small Italian village 100 years ago.

'You are being kept a prisoner by your parents' fear and I daresay you are also a source of cheap labour, which is both selfish and exploitative. If you leave it much longer you will lose your spirit and never make the necessary changes. Stand up to them and tell them that either you have the freedom to live your life by going out and meeting people or you will move away from home. Their fear of "what people will say" will make them give in if you stand firm. I know how hard it will be for you, but if you consider how bleak your future will be if you do nothing, you will find the courage to do what has to be done. It's your life that will be wasted. Is there a priest of your nationality who will back you up and talk to your parents?

'Make a break now, and if a good man of different nationality comes along, don't knock him back because of your parents' wishes. They don't want to lose you as a daughter and will get over their initial bad feelings. Act today and change your life! You owe it to yourself.'

The next letter, from Grazia, was all the more surprising because it arrived in 1990 and showed me that the change in attitude I had observed was not as complete as I thought.

'I am Italian, 18 years old and life is not worth living. My parents are so strict I am not allowed to do anything that other girls do. I am not allowed to talk to boys, or go to discos or wear modern clothes. I'm not even allowed to have girlfriends. I know my parents love me and I love them but what are they afraid I'll do if they give me a little freedom? I've been brought up to know what is right and wrong and I would not do anything to disgrace them or myself. Every time I ask to go anywhere my father slaps me and calls me an awful Italian name and Mum doesn't even stand up for me, but agrees with him. I go to work but if I'm a few minutes late I'm accused of the most terrible things. I've been asked out by a few boys but I always say no as I know I would not be allowed out the door. I am so unhappy. Can you help, Kate?'

'I can understand how unhappy you are and feel sad for you and all the girls from other nationalities who write with this same problem,' I wrote back. 'Second generation migrants such as you are caught in the conflict between two cultures and miss out on the joys of being young in either country. It is fear which motivates your parents' behaviour, fear that you will be exposed to temptation and lose your good name which would reflect badly on them. They keep you in line by caging you in. What they don't realise is that they are clinging to very old customs which have probably even disappeared from the 'old' country.

'It might surprise you to know that I receive letters from Australian girls whose parents are also strict and old-fashioned. So nationality isn't the only criterion for this kind of restriction. I can't tell any of you to defy your parents, but I do urge you to keep at them to extend your boundaries and give you more freedom, even if it means constant fireworks. I urge you to prepare yourself for the future by learning life skills and work skills so that when you are old enough you can leave home and make the life you want. But please don't 'escape' into marriage, will you? You would not have the experience to make a balanced choice and would probably make an unfortunate choice. Try to break this cycle with humour rather than bitterness. Humour works well in any language.'

AN ARRANGED MARRIAGE

Fatima's problem sounded far-fetched in this age and culture, but I knew it was authentic.

'I am 19 and in love with an Australian boy I work with. My parents are from Lebanon and they are furious with me, especially my father. He says he has promised me to a friend from Lebanon who has only just come to this country. My father says if I don't marry this man he will take me back to Lebanon and find me a husband there. My mother cries a lot but she won't go against my father's wishes. I love my boyfriend but I don't dare disobey my father.'

I did not know what to advise. I was aware of the custom of arranged marriages in many countries and knew that statistics showed they often worked out better than marriages based on a passing infatuation. I didn't want to give advice which might be 'right' for Australia but which might jeopardise *her* future.

I felt that if her feelings for her boyfriend were very deep, she would defy her father without any prompting from me. It was not my place to advise defiance. What I did suggest was that she contact a priest of their religion and nationality and talk together before making a decision. I did not hear from her again and can only hope that she found happiness.

CROSS-CULTURAL RELATIONSHIPS

My advice to people interested in forming a relationship with someone of another race is always aimed at removing barriers of race and treating people as people, while recognising the difficulties involved in any inter-racial relationship. Relationships all have their own difficulties to be overcome, but it would be foolish to ignore the unexpected problems posed by differences in culture and background, just as it is foolish to see only the differences and ignore the qualities we all share as members of the human race.

I urge them to be honest and open with each other and with themselves before making a choice, to look into the future and imagine what their lives will be like in five or ten years' time if they marry this or that person. But then, this applies to anyone who is thinking of making a permanent commitment, regardless of race. Racial difference is only one extra challenge to be faced.

Kristine's problem is one I am beginning to see more often.

> 'I am attracted to a young man at work. I've been out
> with him once and feel that I'd like to know him
> better. My problem is that he is Asian. I'm afraid that
> when my parents meet him they won't approve and
> will stop me from going out with him. What can I do?'

'Don't leave it until your parents meet him,' I advised. 'If you do you'll be risking a pointless confrontation.

'The best thing to do is tell them now about your growing friendship for the young man. Concentrate on your wise point — that you'd like to get to know him better. Then ask them to do the same before passing any judgement on the friendship.'

This next letter from Linda has a new twist:

'I am a 16-year-old Australian female. I have been going
with an 18-year-old Turkish male for a week. Already
he won't let me go out or even see my friends. I am
worried because he has a very bad temper.'

My advice was to get out of the relationship quickly.

'I am not racist and I am not saying he is bad, only that the vast
cultural differences will make for a very unhappy, fraught association. But I urge you not to be alone when you tell him it is over,
especially as you say he has a bad temper. Better still, write him
a letter and say your parents don't approve of the friendship.
With his background where parents' wishes are law, he will
accept that reason more readily than your own word. And make
sure he does not waylay you when you are out. Protect yourself
by walking with someone else, either a family member or a
friend. Please note that I would have given exactly the same
advice if your boyfriend had been Anglo-Australian and behaved
in the same way.'

Stephen wrote:

'I have a 17-year-old Italian girlfriend. I am 20 years
old and not Italian. In the three weeks that I have
been going with her, I've seen her a couple of times
and we both love each other. But there is a lot of
interference from her parents. They have this custom
that their daughter should go out with an Italian guy.
I have been trying to get her to go out with me for
three months, and finally succeeded. Now I don't want
her parents stopping the relationship. They are living
with old-fashioned customs and I believe that teenagers
in the nineties are entitled to their freedom. But I'm
afraid of doing the wrong thing.'

'Your talk about being in love after just three weeks, in which
you have seen her only twice, is premature and is bound to turn
her parents against you. Let me assure you that many Australian
parents and teenagers have exactly this same problem so it's not
just a matter of ethnic customs which are getting in your way.
Your best strategy is to behave like a gentleman and convince

them that you won't lead their daughter astray. It won't get you far to be antagonistic with them. They may well be old-fashioned in their attitudes, but their concern for their daughter's welfare is their privilege, and you had better respect it. You are still young and have no experience of life and cannot, therefore, make mature judgements for others. Behave like a gentleman and take the relationship slowly.'

OUR CHILD FEELS 'DIFFERENT'

The next letter was from Sonia and dealt with yet another aspect of cultural differences.

'We came from Lebanon six years ago and are happy in our new country, but our eldest son who is nine has been very unhappy at school and always seems cranky at home. At last he told me the other children made fun of him because he took different lunch food to what they had, and also because he didn't have money to spend at the school canteen. I do not give him money because I always give him healthy food and do not like him to eat rubbish, but I do not want him to be unhappy, so what do I do?'

I told her, 'You are wise to teach your son good eating habits early. However, for the sake of his emotional health, you must compromise a little and allow him an occasional "treat" from the canteen which won't do him any harm. Continually feeling different will hurt him much more.'

WHERE'S 'HOME'?

This next letter from Gianna is one of the most unusual I have received from an emigrant and gives a new slant on what being a migrant really means.

'You will think it strange to get a letter from Italy, but I used to read your page when I was in Australia and liked the answers you gave. I hope you can give me some good advice as I am very unhappy. I am 55,

married with three children and seven grandchildren. I
lived in Melbourne with my husband and children for
25 years but we always talked about going back to
Italy. In 1985 my husband and I came back here to
settle in the town where we were both born. Here we
have brothers and sisters and lots of nieces and
nephews, but our three children are all in Melbourne,
married with their own families. They like it there and
don't want to come back here. For the first few weeks
we were happy to be back, but now I'm heartbroken. I
miss the children and grandchildren and I miss the life
we had there although I had never really accepted it.
Perhaps that was my trouble.

'We have joined a couple of clubs formed by other
migrants who have returned here. One of these clubs is
called the Koala Club and another is the Kangaroo Club.
We get together sometimes and talk about old times in
Australia. We even try to have a barbecue, but it's not
the same. Why do I feel like this when all the time I
was there I longed to be back in my own country? I
miss Australia more than I ever imagined I could.
Please give me some comfort and advice.'

As a mother and grandmother myself, I felt deeply for
Gianna's anguish and wondered what had triggered the decision
to make such a move. The pull of one's native land can be
overwhelming, but her letter also highlighted the problems
which arise from living in the past and in fantasy rather than in
reality. What Gianna had not realised in time was that people
give places a meaning and purpose. Rearing a family puts down
roots which are just as deep and strong as the roots we have in
our place of birth. Her years in Australia where she had formed
her family had created its own bonding.

There was little I could say other than to suggest that she plan
and save for short trips to see her family in Australia. I also
suggested that she keep in touch through letters and as many
phone calls as they could afford. Messages on tapes were also a
good idea, as were photographs.

I urged her to talk things over with her husband and consider
the possibility of coming back to Australia to stay if that was what

they really wanted. I warned her not to be influenced by what other people would tell her, but to follow her heart. I ended by saying that she and her husband were not too old to make a fresh start. If they had learned what they truly wanted from life, their experiences had not been wasted.

A year later I was surprised to receive a letter from Gianna, this time from Melbourne. They had realised, she wrote, that their home was here and that they had felt like foreigners in their place of birth. I felt that this time their decision was a total commitment with no looking back except for the occasional nostalgic memory.

Elenie wrote of the problems this restlessness can have for the other members of the family:

'I am a married woman of 45, have four children and am of Greek origin. I have lived in Australia since I was four. My problem is my father. He has been living with us since my mother died five years ago. We are glad to have him but what is causing a lot of trouble is that he won't settle down either here or in Greece where he has two sisters and a brother. In these five years he has gone back three times. When he is here he is restless and moody. When he is there he writes that he can't wait to get back here. All this is upsetting me, and my husband is beginning to complain. As my father is now 76, I don't want to be unkind or ask him to leave, but it's getting me down. How do I handle this problem so that everybody is happy?'

I knew there was no answer that would make everybody happy. The most Elenie could do was to tell her father how his behaviour was disrupting her family and come to some sort of agreement.

'Your father is feeling the displacement which many people who know and love two countries often feel. There's not much you can do until he makes up his mind. Tell him how unhappy he is making you and how he is affecting your marriage. Perhaps as he grows older he will realise that the people he loves are more important than places. Home *is* where the heart is. It is possible that he will work this restlessness out of his system, and make a decision.

'His behaviour need not disrupt your family — unless you let it. Get him to talk about his feelings. You could even suggest that he write down his reminiscences to hand down some of his past to your children. It would be good therapy for him as well. But above all, keep your relationship with your husband on a loving basis and give him as much attention as you seem to be giving to your father.'

11

Depression, Alcoholism and Other Problems

IN THIS SECTION we have some letters which don't fit neatly into any of the other chapters. Not that we can ever draw a line down the middle of any situation and label it as this or that problem — the symptom and causes always overlap. Often we begin with one difficulty and find as we go along that the core of the problem is something quite different.

FEELING DEPRESSED OR ANXIOUS

In the past few years, letters like the following one from Penny are more and more frequent. It disturbs me that such deep apathy has set in so early. In the past, youth was always synonymous with ideals, enthusiasm and exuberance — what has happened to put out the light?

'In the past two years I have become very pessimistic and sometimes I feel as if I could weep for the whole human race. I go to my job which is considered a good one, mix superficially with people and to all appearances I am living a "normal" life, whatever that is. But inside I feel so empty, as if there's a great big void which nothing and no one can fill. Life to me seems no more than an exercise in futility.'

Penny isn't alone in her feelings of cosmic misery. Most thinking people suffer from occasional attacks of angst, which is the name given to the anxiety brought about by reflection on the

196

human condition. I don't know what causes it, but the feelings of emptiness and futility Penny speaks of often stem from an absence of clearly-defined goals and lack of commitment to anyone or anything beyond her own or her family's immediate needs. Most of us have short-term and long-range goals: to give our children a good education and see them happily leading their own lives; to pay off our mortgage and maybe afford a decent holiday. But commendable as these goals may be, they are limited and lack the importance of other, larger purposes — service to humanity and the social concern which will lead to responsible action.

In order to become fully alive, everyone must have goals which are more than self- or family-centred — they must be larger than life. Our increased awareness of the deprivations and needs of other peoples, our concern for the future survival of our planet are all hopeful signs. Perhaps this is what Penny needs to do: to become intensely committed to some purpose which transcends her own immediate interests. Standing on the sidelines, weeping for the human race is no solution.

Unemployment is an increasing problem which none of us can ignore. I am receiving more and more letters expressing hopelessness and despair. Vicki's letter is only one of many.

> 'I've been out of work for 2½ years and I'm getting
> very depressed about it. I can't understand why I can't
> get a job as a shorthand typist. I live with my mother
> and she's very understanding, but I had a job for nine
> years before I was made redundant. It's hard to get
> used to being on the dole. I feel so demoralised that
> now I'm terrified before an interview. If I'm going to be
> out of work for some time to come — which is how it
> looks — how can I cope with this feeling of being a
> nobody who is no use to anyone?'

'It's the feeling of helplessness which is the hardest to bear, isn't it, so anything you do which will make you feel causative is a good start. Have you any talents you could put to good use from home? Or you could enquire at your Employment Office about adding to your skills or training in a totally different field?

'But on the psychological side, you don't need to wait until you get a job to get that wanted feeling. You can go straight to where you're wanted very badly — and that's to local hospitals, children's homes, homes for the aged and so on where voluntary help is always in short supply. The Volunteers Bureau would be a good place to enquire as to where your talents could best be used to help others. Helping in some caring area of society will do a lot for others and it will restore your purpose in life. You will feel like a 'somebody' again. And although what you do must be done for its own sake and not for financial gain, you'll probably find it easier to get a job through this giving of yourself, than if you sit at home being miserable.'

It is only in recent years that 'panic attacks' as such have been recognised for what they are. With the benefit of hindsight, I realise that many of the 'nervous breakdowns' which I read about in the early seventies were in reality panic attacks. Here is Judy's letter:

> 'For the past three years anything slightly out of
> normal routine has sent me into a state of panic, and
> it's getting worse instead of better. I'm 19 and almost
> certain that I'm experiencing a permanent nervous
> breakdown. Is there any cure? I would appreciate any
> advice that would help me overcome this so that I can
> get on and enjoy my life.'

'Yes, there is a cure and it is easier to apply than you imagine. A few years ago this would not have been the case.

'Get in touch with Dr John Franklin at the School of Behavioural Science, Macquarie University, Sydney 2109, and ask for a Home Programme which includes a diagnostic questionnaire and can be done at any time. This programme is recognised as the best cure for panic attacks. The fee involved is very modest.

'The fact that you feel so positive about life despite your panic attacks means you have a lot going for you and will be able to overcome them.'

Bette's problem — worry — is one that most people suffer from at some stage, but, fortunately, not everyone allows it to take over their lives. When it does, it is as destructive as any major disease — in fact, chronic worry can often precipitate disease by affecting the immune system.

> 'I am a chronic worrier. I tend to blow things out of proportion, brood and create problems that don't exist. I also tend to be very hard on myself and find it hard not to take life too seriously. I am 26 years old and have a good life, and I want to overcome this habit so that I can get on with it and be happy. I have just started to do some relaxation tapes, but could you please give me some further practical advice.'

'Anxiety is generally caused by suppressed emotion — fear, anger or guilt — which has not yet become focused or conscious. It also occurs when we try to escape facing conflicts about important emotional issues in our lives. Your perfectionist attitude which you use to beat yourself with is also damaging. Can you try to be as kind and forgiving to yourself as you would be to a good friend? Each time you have a worrying thought, mentally crumple it up and toss it into the wastepaper basket. Then replace it with some kind thought about yourself — remember something you did well, a compliment paid to you, a talent you know you have, an awareness of others. Mix with lots of friends you like. It does us all good to see ourselves reflected in other people's eyes. It helps us to affirm ourselves. And I suggest that you consider whether your energies are being used to their best advantage. When we are not fulfilled, our energy dams up and lies there, stagnant — a good breeding ground for worry. When you are doing what you love, worry disappears.

'The relaxation tapes are a good start. You might also consider meditation. And a couple of sessions with a psychologist or counsellor would be helpful. You can also write to Dr Franklin at the School of Behavioural Science, Macquarie University, Sydney 2109, and ask for a home programme which will be sent to you for a small fee.

In recent years, depression in young mothers has become so widespread it has earned the name of **Suburban Housewife's Syndrome**. There's no doubt that rearing children is a joyous task but it can also be difficult and unrelenting. The nuclear family, for all its benefits, has cut off many young mothers from the mainstream of life with no emotional or physical back-up which was readily available within the extended family. Perhaps the many choices available to them today have made more mothers dissatisfied with their humdrum routine. Let's look at a few letters on this topic. Clare wrote:

'I love my husband and three young children but lately life is not worth living. I am 25 and held a good job until I married but now I am unable to cope. Everything gets me down — the housework, the children, the never-ending cooking and washing. The doctor just puts me on tablets which make me worse because I am like a zombie and then I fall behind even more and that makes me even more depressed. I feel so lonely and cut off from everything. Surely this is not the way life was meant to be?'

'A great many women feel as you do when they marry and have children and find that where the job they held before took up only a part of their lives, marriage and motherhood involves them totally and without a break. The strain of looking after three little ones will sap anyone's vitality and spirit. What you need is relief from the hopelessly bogged down feeling which comes from the demanding job of rearing children.

'I know you'll say you haven't the time or opportunity for outside interests, but look on it as a prescription for yourself and your marriage. Join a playgroup in your area and get together with other young mothers with small children. Look after someone else's children for half a day and then you can have a half day free when yours are looked after. Try to organise your life so that you can go out one night a week with your husband — it needn't be an expensive outing, even a walk or having a coffee at the local centre can give you a lift. Take up some hobby or interest or sport — there are so many activities available these days, you will be able to choose what you really want. Your local paper, community centre or Baby Clinic will guide you there.

'And throw away your pills. By mixing with other young mothers you will share common experiences so that they become easier to bear. And when you know you have something to look forward to, you seem to whizz through the chores more quickly. No doubt you'll find excuses not to do anything suggested above, but I urge you to think about it and realise that no one can help you except yourself. Once you see that you are not helpless to make things happen the way you want, your life will take on new meaning. Women can be marvellously nurturing and supportive of one another and that is what you need.'

ALCOHOLISM

Alcoholism is a problem I read about in many letters. In the early years of my column such letters nearly always referred to older people. In recent years. younger people who drink too much and find it difficult to give it up, have been writing to me.

Here is Suzie's letter:

'I have lived with my boyfriend who is 31, for the past seven years. I am 35. My boyfriend has always enjoyed drinking with the boys, but over the past two years it has become a real problem. He goes out after work with his mates, rarely phoning me to say where he is, and arriving home at all hours. Often he doesn't come home at all, saying he slept over at a friend's place. When he does come home he's too tired to talk to me and I am lonely, and becoming more and more unhappy. I've tried many times to talk to him and he promises to stop drinking. He will do so for a week — but then he's back to his old habits. I'm tired of being left on my own and am seriously considering leaving and starting a new life. Our relationship is quite one-sided. I am unable to have children but he has three by a previous marriage. They are not living with us and I sometimes think that if I could have a child he might stay home more. Do you think I should leave?'

'In the circumtances, it's just as well you don't have a child,' I replied. 'A child can never hold together a relationship that is beset with so many problems. Your best bet is to contact Al-Anon which is geared to the families of alcoholics. Your boyfriend appears to be an alcoholic. You'll be surprised at the insight and support you'll get by joining this organisation. That is the only way you can help yourself, as well as your boyfriend and the relationship, so don't dismiss it as being irrelevant to you. With their help you'll be able to make a clearer decision about whether to leave or stay. With all the goodwill and intelligence in the world you can't do it on your own, so I strongly urge you to seek this help as soon as possible.'

Pam wrote:

'My husband has a very important job which causes him a lot of stress and strain. So when he's out entertaining business acquaintances he often drinks too much, and when he comes home he says hurtful things to me which he can never remember afterwards. He's usually very kind and generous and we could be happy if it weren't for the pressures on him that make him so cruel to me.'

'Most people's jobs are important to them and we all get stresses and strains of some kind, but we don't all drink too much in order to cope with them,' I said. 'If I were you, I'd stop making excuses for him and persuade him to find other ways of coping with pressure. He could learn to relax more, or spread his interests beyond work to some sport or hobby. He might even be interested in learning to meditate to relieve his tension. If he won't hear of this, and actually prefers to drink too much, then you'd better do as he does and forget the drunken remarks. If his drinking worsens, you should see a counsellor.'

SEXUAL HARASSMENT AT WORK

Sexual harassment is a problem more women than men seem to suffer from. Here is Linda's letter:

'I work in a small business with an amorous boss. He has been having affairs with all the girls, including me. I thought I was the only one for him, but I have found

out that the other girls thought the same. Should we
all gang up on him and tell his wife, or should we
carry on until his wife finds out about all of us?'

'Don't inform his wife,' I wrote. 'She is probably aware of the
sort of man she is married to and will deal with him herself and
in her own way. If you are on good terms with the other girls,
you should talk it over with them. Write a joint letter in which
you tell him how much you dislike what is happening and what
you will expect of him in the future in terms of respect and
consideration. If he threatens to dismiss any of you, tell him that
you will report him to the Anti-Discrimination Board. At the
same time, consider the part you have played in all this and
make up your mind to keep business and sex as separate parts of
your life in the future.'

'We are two girls of 17, working in an office to which a
married man in his mid-40s makes a lot of unnecessary
calls. While he's there he doesn't just stare, he leers
and makes suggestive remarks which we find offensive.
We don't want to leave our jobs, but feel that he'd only
make trouble if we reported him, even though we know
we are within our rights to do so. What advice can you
give us?'

'Unfortunately there's never been a shortage of leering office
Romeos. Just treat his silly remarks as silly and stupid and not
worthy of notice. When he no longer gets a reaction from you
(it's your "flustered" reaction which gives him a buzz), he may
give up his little game as pretty unsatisfying.

'If he doesn't, you can always report him to the Anti-
Discrimination Board.'

WHY HAS MY BEST FRIEND CHANGED?

Cecile wrote:

'A neighbour who has been my best friend for ten
years, has suddenly stopped contacting me. She makes
excuses if I ask her to come and have a cup of coffee

with me, whereas until this change she would welcome
it. If we meet in the street she either pretends she's in
a hurry, or chats for a moment, stiffly, and as if she
can't wait to get away. I can't think why she should
have turned against me. Can you suggest something I
can do to be friends again?'

'Why not try a frank, direct enquiry next time you see her. Ask
her if she is angry with you about anything? This approach will
do equally well if, as is likely, she hasn't fallen out with you but
with life in general, and is unhappy or depressed. Of course, if
she is in a 'low' state of mind it is possible she has felt slighted
by some trivial word or deed which could normally pass unnoticed. If she has never needed your help and sympathy before,
she may now think of herself as a burden if she confides in you.
Show her she is not.'

I WAS A SHOPLIFTER

A problem which crops up occasionally is the one where a
person, usually a woman, has been convicted of shoplifting and
carries the fear and guilt for many years. This letter is from
Hilda.

'Several years ago, I picked up an item in a store and
was charged with shoplifting. I don't know why I did
it as I've never done anything dishonest in my life. I
have been sick with guilt as I have three grown-up
sons and would die if they found out. Now it has
caught up with me. A friend has invited me to go on a
cruise as I've been very ill. My sons think it's
wonderful and are going ahead with arrangements. They
can't understand my hesitation. I've hear that if your
have criminal record you can't apply for a passport.
What can I do?

'You have been worrying yourself ill without any reason. The
Passport Office of the Department of Foreign Affairs assures me
that there is no way your passport would be withheld, or that any
reference would be made on your long-past lapse. There *are*

certain situations where a passport would be withheld, but always in much more serious offences than yours — where there is a warrant out for a person's arrest, for instance, or for someone convicted of possessing drugs. Relax and enjoy your cruise.'

12

The Seven-day Mental 'Diet'

AT THE BEGINNING of this book, I said that what is going on constantly in our minds and heads affects how we perceive the world. We can change our reality by changing our thoughts.

The first step in doing something for ourselves is to look at the negative patterns of our life which are caused by deep-rooted habits of thinking, and substitute new and confident traits.

People who say nobody likes them, that the world is an unfriendly place, are interpreting life in this way because of their fears. They project their own lack of love and trust onto everyone else and it is mirrored in all their relationships.

Once their attitude is transformed to greater acceptance and goodwill towards themselves and their fellow human beings, these same people will smile broadly and remark on how friendly everyone has suddenly become. I have seen this happen again and again in my counselling. It sometimes takes them a while to realise that nothing has changed except the way they are looking at things.

The seven-day mental 'diet' is a recipe for change which I have devised for turning habits which are making us miserable, into a workable, hopeful course of action which will reverse our outlook on life.

How does this mental diet work?

We promise ourselves that just for one week we will cut out completely, unkind, negative thoughts and words. We will consciously pull ourselves up when we think negatively and notice what we are doing. We will not be mean or dishonest, spiteful or envious in thought, word or deed with anyone. No more gossip or snide remarks. We will 'act as if' we are happy, joyful, loving and confident, regardless of how we feel. The American psychologist, William James has said that by acting 'as if' we eventually come to acquire the quality we are pretending to have. We need to train our minds for positive programming, instead of the negative input it has had so far. In this mental diet, we treat everyone with respect and compassion. We become kinder to everyone including ourselves and suddenly the world seems more friendly. It sounds too simple to be true but its results can change our lives around.

As with any diet, it requires effort and our success will be equal to the effort we put into it. It builds up our trust in ourselves and our ability to take charge of our lives. We no longer feel helpless. We can rely on our own word.

The diet consists of daily routines to be followed for a week. We will call them 'mental push-ups'. They begin as soon as we wake up, even before we open our eyes. We look on the day as a new start, another chance, a clean page on which we can write whatever we want. To use an old cliché of the seventies: 'Today is the first day of the rest of my life'. We determine to do better than the day before, but not to get angry with ourselves if we fail. We will release past mistakes and let them go.

Before we get up we fill our minds with simple gratitudes, no matter how small or ordinary. It's good to remember that if we always focus on what we don't have, we will never have enough. If we appreciate what we do have, we stop feeling deprived. Being alive is something to be grateful for, as is even moderate good health. Don't dismiss the pleasures of people you love, and of food, sex and sleep. List the many things you can do — talking, walking, hearing and seeing, rights which many people don't possess. Think of all the advantages you have which were denied to people a hundred years ago, and of the many disadvantaged in the world today. Listing these gratitudes, then, is the first mental push-up which starts off our day.

The second mental push-up is to stand before an open window and breathe deeply. This will increase our oxygen intake and get our circulation going so that we have a feeling of wellbeing. It is much easier to be happy if we are feeling well. But we don't just breathe. There is something we do as well. As we breathe in we imagine we are taking in courage and vitality and enthusiasm. As we breathe out we imagine all the tension, futility and hopelessness flowing from our body. We use this same technique when we are bathing or showering. We watch all our unhappy feelings being washed away with the dead cells and grime on our skin.

The third mental push-up which we do each morning for seven days is this: we look into a mirror and talk lovingly to our image. This may be difficult for many of us but we need to persevere with this particular technique. It will be easier if we imagine the mirror image as being the child-part of ourselves — frightened, discouraged and needy, and that we are the parent who can nurture the fearful, immature part of our self. We talk lovingly to that little child and comfort it. We tell them that they are unique and priceless and that there will never be another like them. This is not conceit, but an acknowledgement and celebration of who we are.

Then we think of anyone who has hurt us or against whom we have a grudge. We forgive them from the heart. We also forgive ourselves for any hurt we have given others.

Now we choose our 'morale-booster' or 'uplifter' — a positive thought for the day. We make up our own, whatever feels right for us. For instance; 'I am whole, free and well', or 'I deserve to be loved', 'I choose to be my own best friend', 'I am relaxed and serene', 'I am peaceful and loving'. We silently repeat this booster at any time through the day when a negative thought intrudes or when we feel we are about to say or do something unworthy. But we must do more than just say the words. We must mean what we say.

The techniques discussed so far are to be used every day. Now I shall set out a specific 'diet' for each of the seven days. As with any diet, you may substitute one suggestion for a similar one which fits in better with your circumstances. For instance, an office worker would have different experiences from a young mother at home, or someone who works full-time, as well as caring for a family. The diet is applied with commonsense according to our lifestyle, age and sex. The only technique which must not be changed is the one where negative thoughts and words are not allowed to settle and multiply, but must always be replaced with a positive, uplifting thought. There is no substitute for that.

DAY ONE

Begin the diet on a Sunday if possible. It will give you time to ease into it. Make this a peaceful day. It is when you are peaceful that your intuition works best. It is also a good way to recharge your batteries. Do the mental push-ups as described. Act as if you are serene. Decide to have a quiet day, alone or with your immediate family or with a quiet friend in a quiet place such as a park or an uncrowded beach. The sight of water is soothing and conducive to gentle thoughts. Or you may decide to potter in the garden. Feel the warmth of the sun and let its rays revitalise you. Close your eyes and let the sun make you feel embraced and nurtured by the universe. Listen to the sounds of nature and relax. At night, listen to music you enjoy. Read something inspirational and savour yet again the quiet pleasures of the day. Be selective about what you watch on TV.

DAY TWO

Do mental push-ups one, two and three. Today 'act as if' you are getting rid of all the clutter in your life and taking charge of what you want to do. Get rid of emotional turmoil such as old hurts and disappointments by writing them down and then crumpling the paper into the wastepaper basket. Or you can think of them and if it is appropriate, punch a pillow or clean out a cupboard, or polish the car — anything which will use up that repressed energy. Tidy up your desk or your drawers or wardrobe and throw out or give away what you no longer need. Getting rid of jumble makes room for good things to flow into your life as well as making you feel you are in charge of it.

As well, today pay a genuine compliment to someone you like and to someone you don't like as much. There is something good we can say about everyone if we look hard enough! Say hello to the bus-driver or the checkout worker at the supermarket. Acknowledge them as human beings. Watch out for negative thoughts such as anger or criticism or impatience which may creep in. Replace them with the booster thought you have chosen. Thank someone for acts of kindness you have taken for granted in the past. Before going to sleep tonight, write down all the good things which made you happy this day. They don't have to be big things. A chat or encouraging word from a friend or colleague, a hug or a posy of weeds from your child, a compliment, a job well-done are all reasons to be joyful. Replay them in your mind as you would a favourite video.

DAY THREE

Mental push-ups one, two and three. Listen to a colleague, a friend or neighbour who needs to talk without you being impatient or dismissive. Be genuinely interested and don't jump in with advice. Just be a sounding board, a channel of healing. If *you* are depressed decide to become consciously active. In depression, energy goes down to zero and needs to be reactivated. The best way to do this is through physical action which is then reflected in your mental outlook. A brisk walk or jog gets the blocked energy moving again and you are no longer bogged down physically and mentally.

DAY FOUR

Mental push-ups. Today, try not to be afraid to say what you honestly think, instead of always agreeing on the surface. If you are feeling frustrated, it could be because you strongly feel the need to say something, yet are afraid to say it. Put your fear to one side and go ahead and say it. Speak the simple truth about how you feel about things. Your honesty will clear the air. Today and every day watch those small negative words and phrases we fall into without being aware of it — phrases such as 'Just my luck!', 'I'm such an idiot', 'Trust me to do the wrong thing', 'Why try?', 'I can't win for losing', 'Isn't it a lousy day?' and all the 'oughts' and 'shoulds' and 'if only's' we say many times in a day without being aware of their cumulative effect. They soon add up and contaminate our deeper thoughts. Imagine them as dead branches on a tree and prune them off.

DAY FIVE

Mental push-ups. Today do some of the things you have been putting off: make that phone call, write that letter, make that appointment with the dentist. Help someone with a chore or job which is not expected of you. Choose a booster statement which affirms you. Refuse to take offence at whatever is said or done just for today. Go for a walk in your lunch-hour and if you catch someone's eye and it is appropriate, smile. Feel at one with the human race. Make a special effort to look bright today — wear a brilliant scarf or a jaunty tie, and choose to spread your good feelings. Think of the negative things you believe about yourself and realise they were probably programmed into your subconscious by significant people and happenings in your life. You don't have to believe them any more. You can erase them from your computer and feed in all the good things about you. Give yourself credit for all your good points and relish your strengths and successes. Write them down and read them again and again.

DAY SIX

Mental push-ups. Today you are free and spontaneous. See yourself as a channel of the life-force which brings good things to you and all who come into contact with you. See your connectedness with all humanity as a bridge which you can cross with joy and pleasure. Give of yourself to anyone who needs you without counting the cost. Become one of those people everyone likes to be with. You do this by being who you really are and not who you think others expect you to be. Don't be afraid to show your vulnerability. When we remove our masks the similarities are greater between us than the differences, and we are all vulnerable. Tonight read something inspirational which touches you deeply. Listen to music you love. Write down all your special gratitudes for the day and savour them.

DAY SEVEN

Mental push-ups. Today believe you can do anything you really desire. Believe in your abilities and visualise yourself as being filled with all the qualities you would like to possess. Know that your relationships are challenges which bring out all that is good in you if they are to work. Congratulate yourself for having kept to this diet. You have reclaimed your power and can trust yourself to do what you say you will do. If you believe in prayer, say whatever uplifting prayers you wish to say. Again make a conscious effort to forgive anyone who needs it and above all forgive yourself for all your negative self-talk in the past.

Reward yourself with any special treats you wish today. A bunch of violets, a record, a book, or some item of clothing — whatever gives you pleasure. Have a massage or a facial, spend time with a loved one or special friend. Decide to keep up at least some of the guidelines of the past seven days. Just as your desire for junk food is diminished after a physical diet, so you will find positive thoughts and nurturing self-talk become more appealing than depressed and negative ones. You will be surprised at how much more you will like yourself and other people, how much lighter you will feel in mind and body. You may find that the one week diet can become a way of life with many bonuses.